Hand
Reflexology

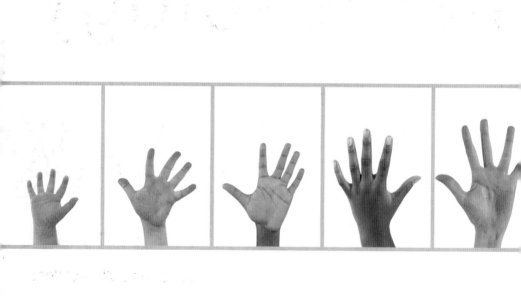

Hand Reflexology

Stimulate your body's healing system

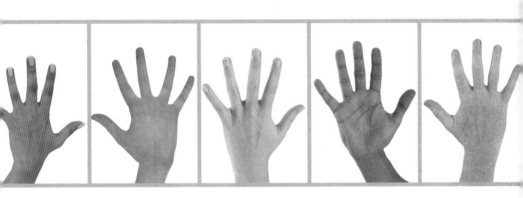

Louise and Michael Keet

hamlyn

A Pyramid Paperback

First published in Great Britain in 2007 by
Hamlyn, a division of Octopus Publishing Group Ltd
2–4 Heron Quays, London E14 4JP

Copyright © Octopus Publishing Group Limited 2007

This material was previously published as *Hand Reflexology*

The right of Louise Keet and Michael Keet to be identified
as the authors of this work has been asserted by them
in accordance with the Copyright, Design and Patents
Act, 1988.

Distributed in the United States and Canada by Sterling
Publishing Co. Inc., 387 Park Avenue South, New York,
NY 10016-8810

ISBN-13: 978-0-600-61593-4
ISBN-10: 0-600-61593-6

A CIP catalogue record for this book is available from the
British Library

Printed and bound in China

10 9 8 7 6 5 4 3 2 1

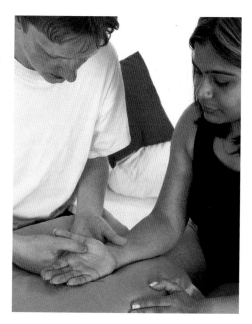

Note: Hand reflexology should not be considered as
a replacement for professional medical treatment: a
physician should be consulted in all matters relating to
health and especially in relation to any symptoms which
may require diagnosis or medical attention. Care should
be taken during pregnancy in the use of pressure points.
While the advice and information in this book are believed
to be accurate, neither the authors nor the publisher can
accept any legal responsibility for any injury sustained
whilst following any of the suggestions made herein.

Dedication
This book is dedicated to Sylvia Keet for her love,
devotion, strength and being the best mother in the
world. And to Hazel Goodwin, former chairman of the
Association of Reflexologists, for her tireless effort in
getting reflexology promoted and giving it its deserved
place in integrated therapies.

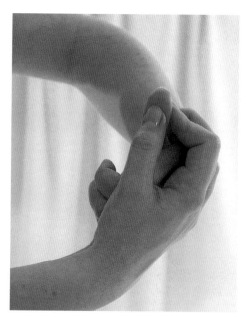

contents

introduction

We all fall ill, whether with a cold, a bad back or something more serious. Consequently we all need healing at some point in our lives. Likewise, I am sure we have all wanted to help a friend or a loved one, but have lacked the skills to do so. Some people help themselves by going to a gym, some see a doctor, others go to a homoeopath or osteopath; some get drunk and some take drugs – but there are other options and reflexology is one of them. Treat this book as a healing bible, a text book, a good read, a reference book or a friend – something to turn to when you or someone you know is in pain.

WHY REFLEXOLOGY?

What is reflexology all about? There are many types of therapies and therapists nowadays and, though they all sound different, they all aim to achieve the same results from their method of healing. Reflexology, like many Eastern therapies, is largely about **energy** and **energy blockages** and balancing a system in 'dis-ease'.

The concept of energy differs in the East. In China, the word *qi*, or *chi* (pronounced 'chee'), means 'vital energy', or 'living force'. In Chinese medicine, *qi* flows along energy channels (meridians) and is crucial to a person's health and vitality. Different types of *qi* exist and they are classified according to their source, location and function. Within the body, there is a link between *qi* and blood because both flow along the same paths. Acupuncture, *qi gong* (a combination of meditation, relaxation, physical movement, mind–body integration and breathing exercises) and *tai chi* (a system of exercises designed to move energies and keep the body strong and supple) all activate the energy currents that flow along the meridians in the body. *Prana* is the Ayurvedic word for *qi*. In the West we often think of our energy as spirit – even Sir Isaac Newton and Samuel Hahnemann (the founder of homoeopathy) recognized the existence of an invisible vital energy upon which good health depends.

Imagine that the reason why we fall sick or fail to get better is because our body systems are blocked and clogged up with waste matter that impedes this flow of energy and needs to be cleared away. The system that produces the waste needs help and this can be achieved with the aid of reflexology.

Reflexology is a therapy which works on this energy by stimulating specific areas in the hands and feet, known as **reflex areas**, that correspond to every part of the body, including organs and glands. The relationship between these areas and parts of the body is the subject of the **zone theory** developed by William Fitzgerald (see page 20).

Treatment of these reflex areas promotes healing in the corresponding part of the body by stimulating the flow of energy and dispersing the blockages that impede energy flow through the body. It is used to relieve stress and tension, improve blood supply, promote nerve conduction and bring about a state of deep relaxation.

WHY HAND REFLEXOLOGY?

Most people associate reflexology with the feet, but hand reflexology has certain advantages. For example, it can be used in situations where there is neither space nor time to work on the feet, and on people who have ticklish feet or are sensitive about having their feet handled. Also, because it is unobtrusive, you can treat yourself in public situations, for example, on an aeroplane, to ward off travel sickness.

Right: Reflex points on the hand can be stimulated to clear energy flows around the body and to treat and prevent a variety of common ailments.

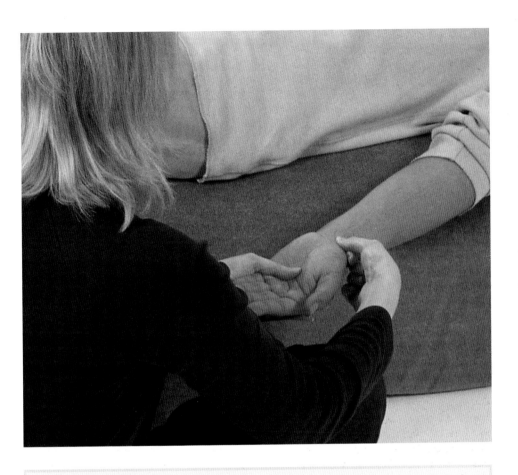

Reflexology: a summary

- Reflexology is based on the concept of energy travelling down zones.
- Reflex areas on the hands and feet correspond to organs, structures and parts of the body.
- Treatment involves applying pressure to these reflex areas.

- Reflexology unblocks energy channels and increases energy levels.
- Reflexology stimulates the body's own healing mechanisms.
- Reflexology balances structures within the body on all levels.

WHY IS REFLEXOLOGY SO POPULAR?

Reflexology is becoming increasingly popular for a number of reasons.

- **Increasing media interest:** More and more articles on reflexology, ranging from its benefits to explanations of the therapy and its efficacy, are being published.
- **Growing attention from the medical profession:** In the UK, many physicians are using reflexology in their practices and clinics, and hospitals, such as University College Hospital in London, are utilizing reflexologists as an economical therapy.
- **Research trials:** Controlled trials are now being carried out in Europe and the USA (see pages 12–13).
- **Government regulation of reflexology:** Worldwide, this is evident in the introduction of training standards and of recognized reflexology qualifications.
- **Improved standards of training:** It now takes a minimum of nine months to train part-time to become a reflexologist.

WHO CAN REFLEXOLOGY HELP?

Reflexology can help almost anyone, but here are some guidelines.

- **The elderly:** Any form of touch benefits the senior citizens in our society. These benefits are huge and, because reflexology works on several different levels, include improved circulation and increased mobility. A person whose mood is improved is more likely to go out or feel better within his/herself. Using hand reflexology is also easier and requires less delicacy than working on the feet.

- **Children:** Gentle reflexology on the hands provides reassurance and comfort to a child. Teenagers can benefit from the de-stress aspect of hand reflexology and from the help with the effects of hormonal changes around puberty. Regular hand reflexology treatments can also enhance the bond between a parent and their child.
- **Babies:** Reflexology can help a baby to release tension after birth and adjust to life in the outside world.
- **People with acute conditions:** Examples include the effects of injury, perhaps from an accident; toothache; a flare-up of an existing condition, such as an arthritic 'episode'; fever and breathlessness. Reflexology can help reduce inflammation, conserve energy and stimulate internal organs, encouraging them to function more effectively.
- **People with chronic conditions:** Some conditions persist for a long time – chronic hepatitis, for example, can last for six months or longer – and there may be little change in the symptoms from day to day. A person who has recovered from the immediate effects of a stroke may experience further deterioration, such as loss of feeling or shooting pains in the limbs. Reflexology can help with the side-effects of medication.
- **Friends and family:** Reflexology is an accessible form of therapy and can be practised virtually anywhere. It is great as either a one-off or a continuing treatment for loved ones and it costs nothing to give. Reflexology also acts as a preventive therapy by detoxifying the body and helping to release the build-up of tension that is associated with stress and stress-related conditions, such as high blood pressure, migraine and chronic neck or back pain.

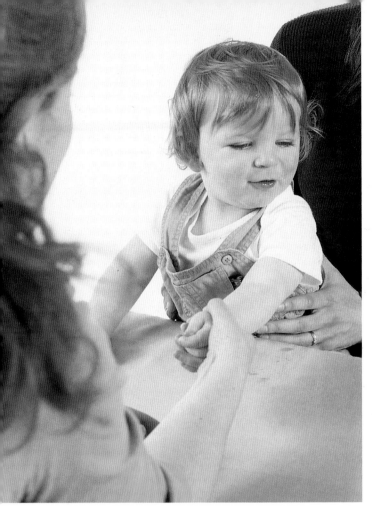

Left: *Babies respond very well to gentle hand reflexology as they are highly receptive to touch. Daily treatments of light massage can give your baby a sense of safety, wellbeing and balance.*

Reflexology: the benefits

- Relaxation – calms the system, giving total physical and mental relaxation.
- Pain relief – has an anaesthetic effect on nerve supply.
- Improved circulation of blood and lymph.
- Boosts the immune system – stimulates the body's own healing system.
- Stress relief.
- Stimulates organs to work efficiently.
- Detoxification – rids the body of waste products and toxins.
- Boosts energy levels.
- Psychological comfort.
- Recovery after injury or surgery.
- Assisting the release of past trauma.
- Human interaction and touch.

HISTORY OF REFLEXOLOGY

Reflexology has been used as an effective healing tool for over five thousand years. As long ago as 2330 BC in Ancient Egypt people believed that stimulating specific areas on the hands and feet would replenish the entire body. However, no single culture has claimed to have discovered this archetypal form of therapy.

The Ancient Egyptians perceived the human body as a symphony of vibrations in which the internal organs represented an intricate orchestra and could be played by stimulation of points in the hands and feet. Before mummification of a body, the soles of the feet were removed in order to liberate the soul from the physical body and from the earth.

Other civilizations that have a long history of pressure-point therapy include those of India, China and Japan. Native Americans were also using this type of therapy for centuries before North America was discovered by Europeans. They believed that the earth held an energy which connected them both physically and spiritually to the earth; illness created disharmony and impeded the free flow of this special energy between them and the earth, so they used the technique to correct this imbalance and to bring about healing.

US president John Garfield (1831–81), who suffered from severe pain following an assassination attempt, also favoured hand reflexology as his main source of treatment.

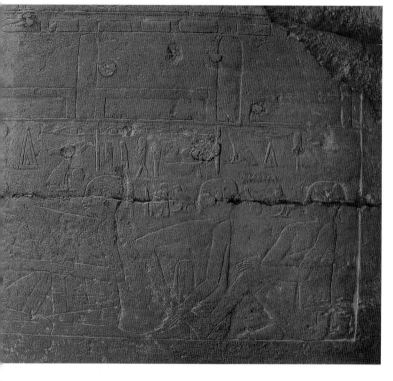

Left: The Ancient Egyptians believed that internal organs could be stimulated through points in the hands and feet. This scene from a pictograph at Saqqara (2500–2350 BC) depicts people massaging feet.

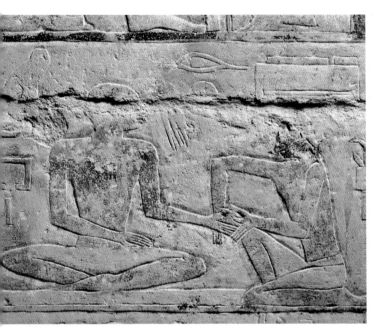

MODERN REFLEXOLOGY

The true pioneer of reflexology was **Dr William Fitzgerald** (1872–1942), an American laryngologist. He was no doubt aware that the Native Americans used a form of pressure-point therapy and, when carrying out minor surgery, he would get his patients to grip combs in their hands in order to block out the pain; wooden clothes pegs on the fingertips and elastic bands around the fingers were equally effective. He also used reflexology successfully to treat morning sickness in pregnant women by squeezing the first and second zones on the dorsal aspect of the hand. Unfortunately the medical profession found his methods time-consuming and, with the advent of general anaesthetics, superfluous.

In 1917, Fitzgerald published a book on **zone therapy**, in which he discussed the link between the palmar surface of the hands and pain in the back of the body, and the dorsal surface of the hands with pain in the front of the body. He was also the first person to chart the zones of the body (see also page 20).

The word 'reflexology' was devised by **Eunice Ingham** (1897–1974), who was known as 'the mother of reflexology'. She was a physiotherapist who used reflexology in her treatments. Eunice lectured extensively in the USA and ran courses teaching others her method of reflexology. However, at that time, reflexology was regarded with suspicion and she was arrested on more than one occasion for practising it without a licence – and that was in 1968!

Nowadays, reflexology is a large part of many people's lives and is the first choice of treatment for a variety of conditions. As a result, more and more people are learning about this valuable form of healing.

CLINICAL EVIDENCE

In the last decade or so, a number of investigations have been conducted in both Europe and the USA into the beneficial effects of reflexology on a variety of conditions.

DANISH STUDIES

In Denmark a great number of clinical studies have been conducted into the effectiveness of reflexology as a treatment. Here are summaries of just a few:

Chronic constipation

In 1991, a study held at the FDZ (Danish Reflexology Association) Sealand local branch on 20 women aged between 30 and 60 years showed an increase in the average frequency of bowel movements from 4.1 to 1.8 days.

Absenteeism

Over a three-year period up to 1992, 235 post-office workers were treated with reflexology for a number of health problems. Of these, 170 reported a good effect, 60 some effect and five no effect. Absenteeism was reduced from 11.4 to 8.5 days per person per year, representing an enormous saving to the company.

Migraine

In the early 1990s, it was estimated that headaches were responsible for the annual loss of three million working days and were the most common complaint among the adult population. As a result, in 1995, the National Board of Health, the council concerned with alternative treatment, the Department of Social Pharmacy and the Royal Danish University of Pharmacy conducted a nationwide study on headaches.

The study involved 220 people who were experiencing chronic headaches and 78

reflexologists who held a series of reflexology treatments over a three-month period. At the beginning of the treatment programme, a physician checked each patient in order to confirm the headache diagnosis. Each patient kept a headache diary, from which the evidence was collated, and each completed a questionnaire. Qualitative interviews were conducted at the end of the treatment sessions. Results showed that 81 per cent were either cured or helped and 19 per cent dispensed with drugs.

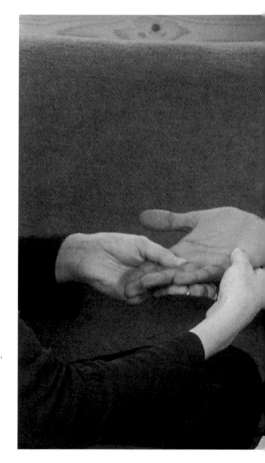

Primary health problems and return for treatment

In 1995, the municipality of Aarhus, Denmark, employed three reflexologists, who treated 143 patients over a six-month period. Of these patients, 79 per cent were either cured or greatly helped with their primary health problem. In addition, 57 per cent were helped with secondary problems, 30 per cent became more satisfied with their jobs, and 92 per cent wanted to continue having reflexology.

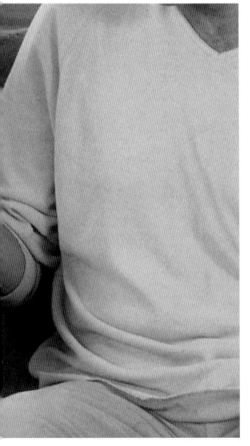

Birth

In 1998, at Gentofte Hospital in Copenhagen, 61 of 68 women who received reflexology treatment prior to giving birth reported a positive pain-killing effect during delivery. Of 14 women with retention of the placenta, 11 avoided surgery.

AMERICAN STUDIES

Clinical studies in America have shown how regular reflexology treatment can benefit the whole body and state of mind.

Premenstrual syndrome

In 1991, Bill Flocco, who founded the American Academy of Reflexology with Dr Terrence Oleson, Associate Professor of Research at the University of California, conducted a study of the effects of reflexology in alleviating premenstrual syndrome (PMS). Results indicated a 62 per cent reduction of PMS in those undergoing reflexology.

Anxiety and pain

Dr Ray Wunderliche, Jr, of Florida notes that reflexology is helpful for people with hypertension, anxiety or pain. Another study, by the School of Nursing, East Carolina University, which reported in 2000, examined the effects of reflexology on anxiety and pain in patients with cancer. All patients received 30-minute treatments and results showed that all the women experienced a dramatic decrease in anxiety and that those with breast cancer felt a decrease in pain. Researchers concluded that reflexology has a place alongside conventional medical care among such patients.

Left: A great number of clinical studies have been conducted into the effectiveness of reflexology. As demand for integrated therapies grows, many countries are beginning to recognize their worth.

how does reflexology work?

There are a number of theories behind reflexology – these relate to the nervous system, pain and its perception, endorphins, energy flow, therapeutic touch, circulation, the placebo effect and, most important of all, the zone theory.

This chapter introduces the reflex points of the hand and maps how they relate to the body. There is an overview of anatomy and physiology of the body, which is essential to understand disorders of the body and how reflexology can help.

the theories behind reflexology

It may be some time before there is a scientific explanation of any of the theories concerning the working of reflexology. Until then, it is important to bear in mind that reflexology works regardless of the how and why. It also works on different levels and no two treatments will be the same, just as no two people are the same.

PAIN THEORY

In order for us to fully explain and understand reflexology, we must first grasp the concept of pain. (At this point it may be helpful to refer to the section on the **nervous system**, see page 32.) The skin (and blood vessels) contains thousands of nerve endings which are specialized to respond to different types of stimuli, such as cutting, pricking or heat, or warning stimuli, such as stretching or pressure. Pain receptors in the body warn of possible injury or caution against repeating an unwise action, such as burning a finger by touching a hot stove. When an injury occurs, signals pass along the nerve pathways to the central nervous system where they are then processed.

Pain thresholds and pain perception

Anxiety and fear are both common emotions that are associated with pain, and pain thresholds, which vary enormously from person to person, are largely associated with these emotions. For example, the pain associated with cancer may seem more intense because it is linked to the fear of death, unlike the pain of indigestion. Any pain always seems worse before the cause is diagnosed and this is all down to perception. In some cases people prepare psychologically for the onset of pain – for example, a sportsman working through a cramp, or a woman about to give birth. Past experience may modify pain perception because of coping mechanisms that

act to reduce pain when it occurs again. Many people learn to cope with pain, but this may cause further problems in another area of the body, which becomes disturbed, unbalanced and in disharmony. Some, finding that conventional medicine does not work, turn to integrated therapies, such as hand reflexology.

Referred pain

Pain felt in a place other than the original site of injury or diseased area is known as **referred pain**. This occurs because the sensory nerves

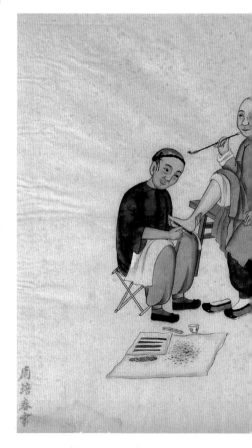

converge before they enter the brain, creating confusion about the true source of the pain. Examples are the toothache that is felt in the ear because both tooth and ear share the same nerve supply, and that from the gall bladder which is felt in the region of the shoulder blade.

ENDORPHIN RUSH

'Endorphin' is a shorterned way of saying 'endogenous morphine'. In the early 1970s, it was discovered that morphine (a pain-killing drug) acted on specific receptor sites (opiate receptors) that are found in some nerve endings in the brain and spinal cord. This discovery led to the identification of the protein-like substances which are now known as **endorphins**. These have an analgesic effect and are thought to be related to mood and stress. They are reported to be at least five times more powerful than morphine. Reflexology stimulates the production of endorphins by clearing nerve pathways that have become overloaded with sensory information.

A good analogy is to think of the reflexologist as an electrician who mends a fuse in the basement in order to fix the light in the attic. In this case, reflexology actually improves nerve stimulation to a particular organ or body part by encouraging it to work efficiently – by balancing itself or reducing the level of toxins – thus normalizing its function.

ENERGY THEORY

The concepts of an electromagnetic circulation and the Eastern theory of *qi* (see page 6) are the basis of the energy theory – the existence of a blueprint or life force invisible to the human eye. The theory goes on to say that energy travels down channels **(meridians)** which facilitate this energy flow. Stress or illness hinders this flow, misaligning the energy signals. The application of reflexology, like acupuncture, realigns this signal and creates a free flow of energy throughout the body.

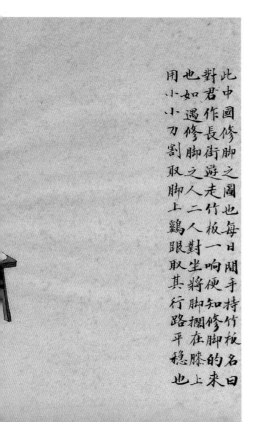

Left: Reflexology is an age-old therapy for stimulating energy circulation. For centuries, the Chinese have advocated the healing power of massage.

THERAPEUTIC TOUCH

The concept of **therapeutic touch**, or 'healing hands', was developed in the USA in 1971 by Dr Dolores Krieger and her mentor, the late Dora Kunz, who was a widely respected healer. Together they originated a non-religious, secular form of healing which combined the laying on of hands with a number of bioenergetic techniques. This technique was then taught at New York University as an extension to the nursing course.

When considering therapeutic touch and its benefits, it is important to bear in mind that the 'laying on of hands' is an ancient practice. It is depicted in Stone Age art, and many references in the New Testament of the Bible refer to the hand as a channel for divine energy and healing. In the Middle Ages, it was thought that the touch of a king's hand would heal the sick, although this is more likely to have been a case of 'placebo healing'.

The theory is that, by touching and stimulating, an exchange of energy takes place between giver and receiver, thus setting the healing process in motion. Healers certainly exist and they have effected many unexplained cures. Therapeutic touch is used widely in hospitals and hospices.

CIRCULATION THEORY

The heart pumps a continuous flow of blood through the blood vessels, providing the cells of the body with oxygen and nutrients and removing the waste products that build up in the system and cause 'dis-ease' and imbalance. As a result, to quote Eunice Ingham, 'Circulation is life, stagnation is death'. Think about this for a moment. Stress causes tension in the cardiovascular system, restricting blood flow and resulting in a sluggish circulation. Therefore, this

Rapport

The ability to establish a rapport with a wide range of people is an important attribute in life, particularly in the field of reflexology. Rapport skills are largely instinctive and are most often found in individuals who are genuinely interested in other people. These skills can be learnt using simple techniques, but a positive mental attitude towards health is a good starting point.

theory argues, waste particles accumulate in the hands and feet, impeding the blood flow, and the build-up of these particles causes stagnation. Because the hands and feet are furthest away from the heart, hydrostatic pressure and gravity (which cause pooling of heavy particles in the feet) intensify this build-up.

During stimulation, this build-up is felt as **adhesions** – fibrous tissue that accumulates like scar tissue. Practitioners speak of these adhesions as crystals, or **crunchified** areas, which cause blockage. These extend all along the fingers or toes and pass directly through the areas of the body that are in distress. Reflexology breaks down these deposits, improving the circulation so that the blood can cleanse the body of these wastes. The waste passes to the lungs, bowel or skin, where it is excreted, which is why it is advisable to drink plenty of water after treatments.

A similar argument suggests that these adhesions are calcium deposits that have settled beneath the skin surface at the nerve endings and created blockages.

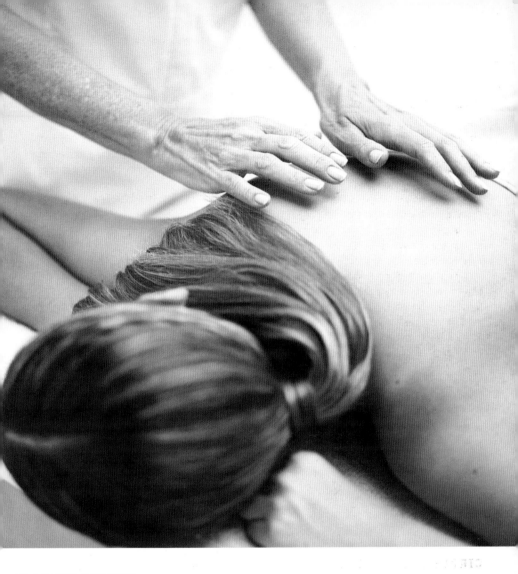

PLACEBO THEORY

The **placebo effect** is the ability of a neutral substance to cure an ailment. This may take place immediately or over a period of time. As an example, some physicians prescribe sugar pills to their patients, whose conditions dramatically improve purely because the patients believe that they will do so. However, this is largely to do with the rapport between the therapist and the patient, and with the power of suggestion.

Above: Healers treat with a laying-on of hands, their hands touching or held just away from the body. The exchange of energy between healer and patient can spark the recovery process.

ZONE THEORY

William Fitzgerald developed the **zone theory** after discovering that he could induce numbness and alleviate certain symptoms in the body by applying pressure to specific points on the hands and mouth.

Zone theory is based on the concept of the body being divided into ten longitudinal zones, extending from the head through to the fingers and toes. There are five zones on each side of the body, passing through the fingers and toes. The left side of the body corresponds to the left hand and foot, and the right side corresponds to the right hand and foot.

Each zone encompasses various parts of the body, the head having five zones on each side. On the hand, the thumb lies in zone 1, the index finger in zone 2, the middle finger in zone 3, the ring finger in zone 4 and the little finger in zone 5.

Energy pathways

Energy travels through the zones and thus there is an **'energy' connection** between all organs, muscles, blood supply, nerve cells and different tissue types along the zones. Disturbance in any part of the body will have an effect on the functioning of any organ or structure within that particular zone.

Applying pressure to the hands and feet will stimulate the flow of energy throughout the corresponding zone of the body; this is because the hands and feet are at the ends of the zones where the reflexes are most sensitive.

The zones

Applying pressure to the hands and feet will stimulate the flow of energy throughout the corresponding zone. The longitudinal zones extend through the body from head to toe and from front to back.

The thumb lies in zone 1

The index finger lies in zone 2

The middle finger lies in zone 3

The ring finger lies in zone 4

The little finger lies in zone 5

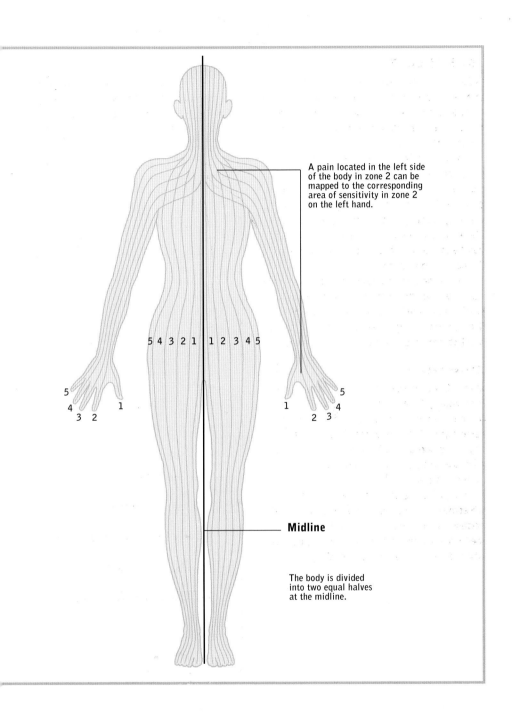

A pain located in the left side of the body in zone 2 can be mapped to the corresponding area of sensitivity in zone 2 on the left hand.

5 4 3 2 1   1 2 3 4 5

5
4   1
3 2

1   5
      4
2 3

Midline

The body is divided into two equal halves at the midline.

reflexology and the hand

ASPECTS OF THE HAND

The photographs below demonstrate the various aspects of the hand (dorsal, palmar, lateral and medial). This may be of help when you come to the section on techniques.

REFLEX POINTS

These points, which are shown on the maps opposite, relate to various parts of the body. They are the basis of any reflexology treatment and it is essential to learn their positions and to know which moves to use when stimulating them.

Dorsal aspect

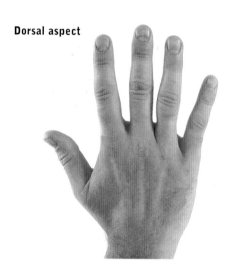

Palmar aspect

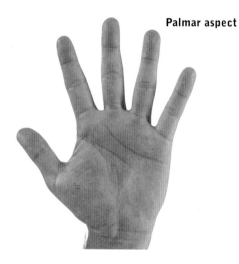

Lateral aspect

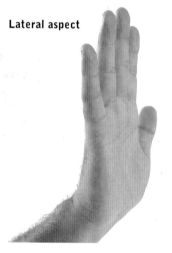

Medial aspect

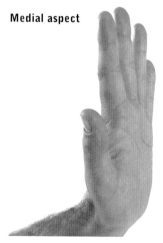

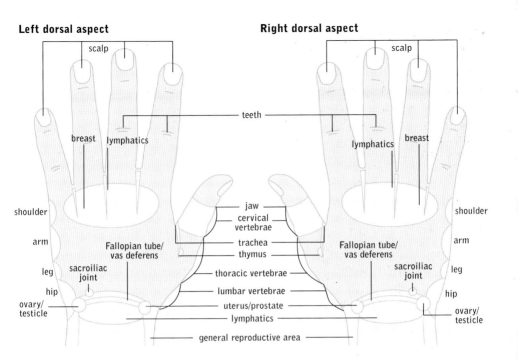

Left dorsal aspect

scalp

breast lymphatics

teeth

shoulder

arm

leg

hip

ovary/ testicle

sacroiliac joint

Fallopian tube/ vas deferens

jaw
cervical vertebrae
trachea
thymus
thoracic vertebrae
lumbar vertebrae
uterus/prostate
lymphatics

general reproductive area

Right dorsal aspect

scalp

lymphatics breast

shoulder

arm

leg

hip

ovary/ testicle

sacroiliac joint

Fallopian tube/ vas deferens

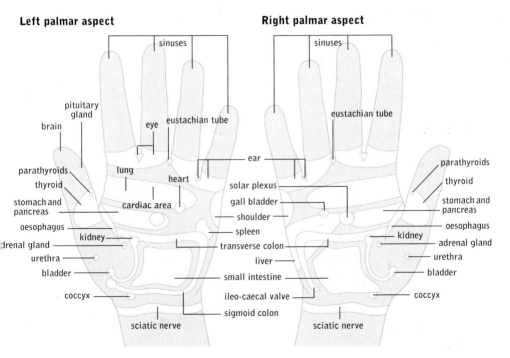

Left palmar aspect

sinuses

pituitary gland

brain

eye eustachian tube

parathyroids

thyroid

lung

stomach and pancreas

oesophagus

adrenal gland

urethra

bladder

coccyx

kidney

heart

cardiac area

sciatic nerve

ear

solar plexus
gall bladder
shoulder
spleen
transverse colon
liver
small intestine
ileo-caecal valve
sigmoid colon

Right palmar aspect

sinuses

eustachian tube

parathyroids

thyroid

stomach and pancreas

oesophagus

kidney adrenal gland

urethra

bladder

coccyx

sciatic nerve

cross-reflexes

Cross-reflexes are points or areas on one part of the body which **'reflect'** another part of the body; the upper limbs, for example, reflect the lower limbs. Other examples are:

- Fingers/Toes
- Hand/Foot
- Wrist/Ankle
- Arm/Leg
- Elbow/Knee
- Shoulder/Hip

Cross-reflexes work on the principles of Dr Fitzgerald's **zone theory** (see page 20), whereby Dr Fitzgerald put clothes pegs on the fingers to anaesthetize parts of the foot.

As an example, consider the pain of tennis elbow in the right arm. You can relieve the pain by imagining the right hand to be the affected elbow and stimulating the corresponding reflexes on the hand. You can also treat that area by working on the matching limb on the right leg, which is the knee. Stimulating the cross-reflex can clear the energy path to the pain and ease movement of the elbow.

It is therefore possible to treat a person with an injury to the toes, foot or ankle by stimulating the corresponding reflex – that is, the fingers, hand or wrist. Conversely, you can stimulate cross-reflexes on the body if you are unable to treat the hand because it is injured.

Cross-reflexes

Reflexes on the limbs are referred to as cross-reflexes (working across from one limb to the other on the same side). When treating a specific ailment you can work that area both on the hand and on the corresponding part of the body.

The arms are reflected by the legs.

The shoulders are reflected by the hips.

The elbows are reflected by the knees.

The wrists are reflected by the ankles.

The hands are reflected by the feet.

The fingers are reflected by the toes.

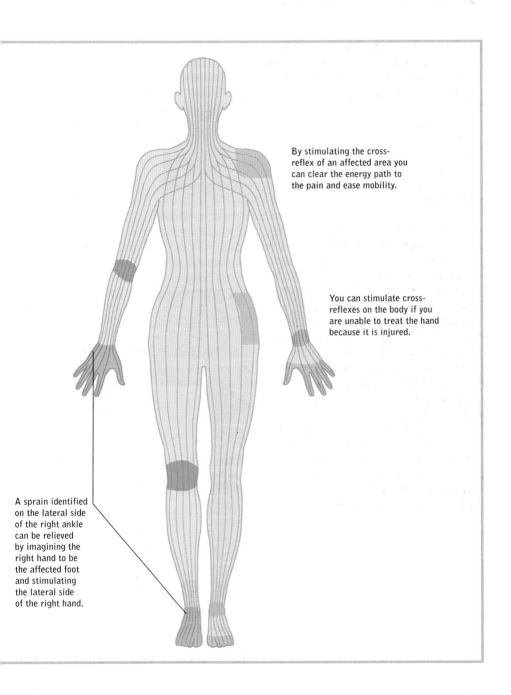

By stimulating the cross-reflex of an affected area you can clear the energy path to the pain and ease mobility.

You can stimulate cross-reflexes on the body if you are unable to treat the hand because it is injured.

A sprain identified on the lateral side of the right ankle can be relieved by imagining the right hand to be the affected foot and stimulating the lateral side of the right hand.

anatomy and physiology of the body

To fully appreciate the effects of reflexology, it is important to understand the structure and workings of the body and its vital systems. These are presented in the form of illustrations and basic descriptions of the functions of their component parts. The section concludes with a detailed description of the anatomy of the hand.

CELL TYPES

The cell is the basic unit of life and is the smallest structure able to perform all the processes that form and define life, such as respiration, movement, digestion, excretion, reproduction and growth. However, many cells of the human body lost some of these abilities when they became specialized for particular functions; for example:

- Nerve cells (**neurones**) transmit nerve impulses.
- Red blood cells (**erythrocytes**) carry oxygen around the body.
- Bone cells (**osteocytes**) lay down bone.
- Secretory cells produce substances that are essential for various body processes; for example, enzymes aid digestion.

The principal parts of the cell are:

- The **cell membrane**, which controls the passage of gases, nutrients and waste matter into and out of the cell.
- The **nucleus**, the powerhouse of the cell, which controls all its functions.
- The **cytoplasm**, which forms the bulk of the cell.

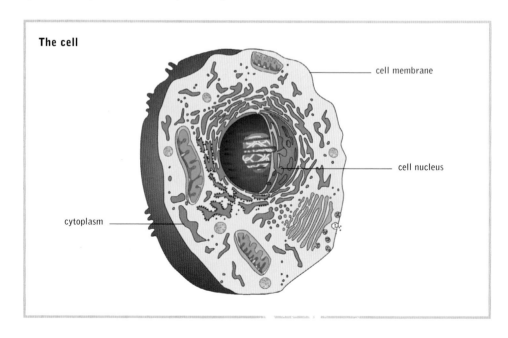

The cell

cell membrane

cell nucleus

cytoplasm

THE SKIN

The skin, the outer covering of the body, is the largest of the body's organs and consists of an outer layer of flattened cells (the **epidermis**) and an inner layer (the **dermis**). These layers contain various structures, each with a specific function; for example:

- The **epidermis** protects against injury and harmful substances and heals sites of injury. It also produces melanin (giving a suntan) to protect against the sun's harmful rays.
- The **blood capillaries**, by contracting when it is cold and dilating when it is hot, regulate body temperature.
- The **nerve endings** are sensitive to both temperature and touch.

- The **hairs** and their muscles also regulate temperature by producing shivering and 'goose pimples' when it is cold.
- The **sweat glands** produce a secretion that cools the body.

In addition, specialized glands **(milk glands)**, unique to mammals, produce milk in order for them to nurture their offspring.

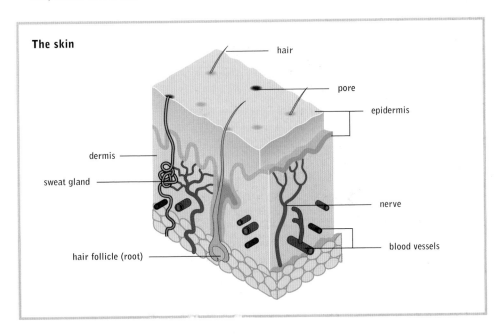

The skin

hair

pore

epidermis

dermis

sweat gland

nerve

blood vessels

hair follicle (root)

BONES

There are exactly 206 bones in the adult human skeleton; 26 in each foot and 27 in each hand. The functions of the skeleton are:

- To support the body, which it does in a similar way to the supports in a high-rise building, with the plaster resembling the muscles and the heating and water supplies resembling the blood system.
- To provide an attachment for the ligaments and tendons, so that the body can move.
- To protect essential organs; the rib cage, for example, protects the heart and lungs and the skull protects the brain.
- To produce red and white blood cells.

MUSCLES

The muscles make up about half the body weight. There are three main types:

1 Skeletal muscle, consisting of banded fibres bound in bundles by connective tissue. These bundles are linked to bones by tendons. Skeletal muscles are largely under our control (reflex actions, such as the 'knee jerk', are an exception) and tend to work in pairs: when one of the pair contracts, the other relaxes, and vice versa.

2 Smooth muscle, described as involuntary as it is not under our conscious control. It consists of elongated cells bound by connective tissue and is capable of slow, sustained contraction. Examples include the muscles of the gut and bladder. It also occurs around the blood vessels and in the skin.

3 Cardiac muscle, a unique muscle, the size of a grapefruit, found only in the heart. It falls halfway between skeletal and smooth muscles. It contracts rhythmically and never gets tired.

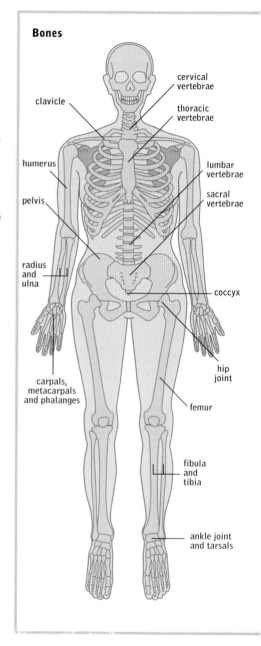

Bones

cervical vertebrae
clavicle
thoracic vertebrae
humerus
lumbar vertebrae
pelvis
sacral vertebrae
radius and ulna
coccyx
carpals, metacarpals and phalanges
hip joint
femur
fibula and tibia
ankle joint and tarsals

Muscles

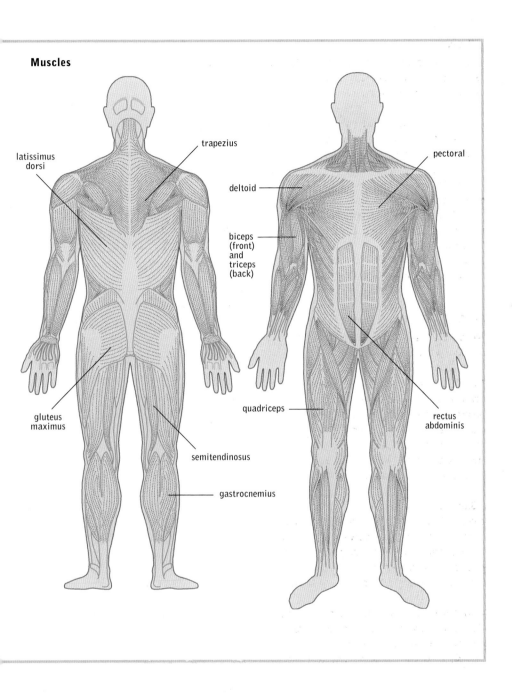

latissimus dorsi

trapezius

deltoid

biceps (front) and triceps (back)

pectoral

gluteus maximus

quadriceps

rectus abdominis

semitendinosus

gastrocnemius

CIRCULATORY (CARDIOVASCULAR) SYSTEM

There are three components of the cardio-vascular system:

1 The heart, a grapefruit-sized organ made of cardiac muscle (see page 28), drives the circulation. It is divided into four chambers:
- **The right atrium and ventricle**, which receive deoxygenated blood from the body and pump it to the lungs (the pulmonary circulation).
- **The left atrium and ventricle**, which receive oxygenated blood from the lungs and pump it around the body (the systemic circulation).

2 The blood vessels: there are three main types:
- **The arteries**, which carry oxygenated blood.
- **The veins**, which carry deoxygenated blood.
- **The capillaries** – small blood vessels that provide a link between the arteries and veins.

3 The blood, consisting of:
- **The plasma**, the liquid part.
- **The red blood cells**, which contain a pigment (haemoglobin) that carries the oxygen or carbon dioxide.
- **The white blood cells**, which fight infection (see Lymphatic system, page 31).
- **The platelets**, which aid the clotting process.

The main functions of the system are:
- Transport of oxygen and nutrients to the cells and carbon dioxide and waste products from the cells.
- Regulation of the body's water content, temperature and pH balance.
- Protection against injury and infection.

By stimulating circulation, reflexology boosts the body's oxygen supply, which enhances energy levels and healing and waste removal.

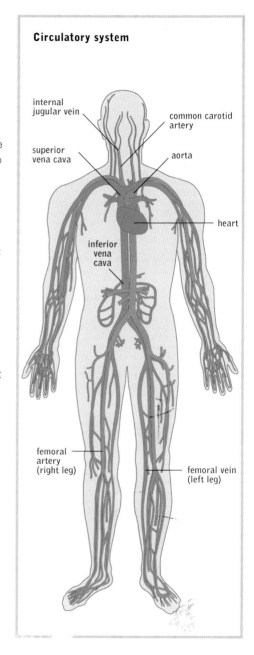

Circulatory system

internal jugular vein

common carotid artery

superior vena cava

aorta

heart

inferior vena cava

femoral artery (right leg)

femoral vein (left leg)

LYMPHATIC SYSTEM

The lymphatic system is one of the most important human body systems and defends the body from foreign bodies such as viruses, bacteria and fungi. Its network of vessels branch through all parts of the body carrying a colourless liquid known as **lymph**, which also returns excess tissue fluid to the circulation and helps combat infection.

The lymph system consists of:

- **Vessels and ducts**, which are responsible for collecting excess lymph and returning it to the bloodstream.
- **Glands**, which produce white blood cells to combat infection.

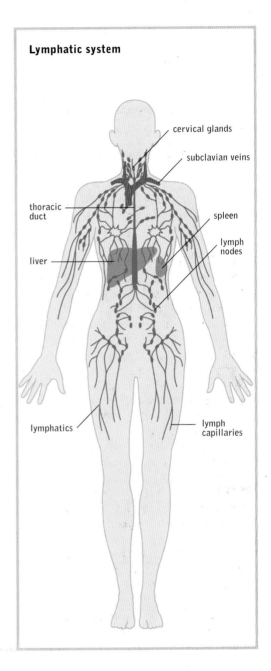

Lymphatic system

- cervical glands
- subclavian veins
- thoracic duct
- spleen
- liver
- lymph nodes
- lymphatics
- lymph capillaries

Swelling of the lymph glands

When producing white blood cells to combat infection, the lymph glands may swell. For example, a bacterial infection in the hand may spread, resulting in a painful swelling in the lymph gland of the armpit. If not treated with antibiotics, it can lead to blood poisoning (septicaemia).

NERVOUS SYSTEM

There are two principal components of the nervous system:

1 The central nervous system, consisting of the **brain** and **spinal cord**, can be likened to a central computer unit that receives, processes and acts on information from sense organs throughout the body. The brain is the control centre where higher processes, such as thinking, decision-making and initiating and controlling actions, take place. Sensory information from the eyes, ears and nose (taste and smell) are carried directly to the brain.

2 The peripheral nervous system, the network of nerve cells throughout the body, provides the link between the central nervous system and the organs and tissues. These links may be unconscious (autonomic) and concerned with functions such as urination or sweating, or conscious (somatic) and concerned with the smooth functioning of the organs and glands.

The **nerve cells** (neurones) are one-way systems, carrying either sensory information or instructions to act. In simple terms, each consists of:

- **A cell body**.
- **A receptor**, which receives sensory information.
- **A transmitter**, which transmits instructions to act.
- **The axon**, a long, spindly fibre, which carries the information or instructions.

Impulses are carried across the junctions (synapses) between receptors and transmitters by a chemical known as a **neurotransmitter**.

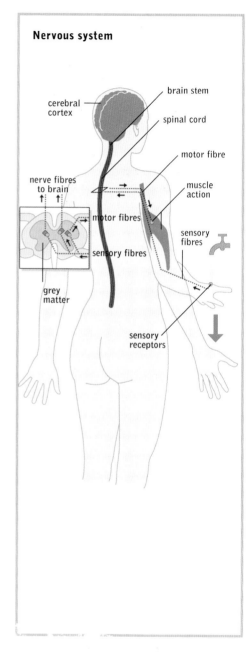

Nervous system

brain stem

cerebral cortex

spinal cord

motor fibre

muscle action

nerve fibres to brain

motor fibres

sensory fibres

sensory fibres

grey matter

sensory receptors

ENDOCRINE SYSTEM AND HORMONES

The endocrine system consists of a group of **endocrine (ductless) glands,** which produce secretions that pass directly into the bloodstream (unlike the secretions of other glands, such as sweat glands, which are passed into ducts).

These secretions, called **hormones,** are basically chemical messengers that affect other organs and glands of the body, stimulating them into action – for example, digestion, energy use, emotion, reproduction and menstruation. In many ways, the endocrine system acts rather like the nervous system.

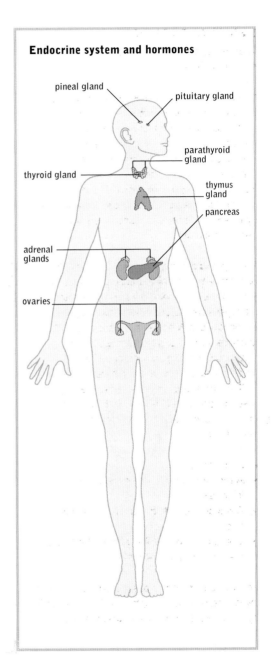

Endocrine system and hormones

pineal gland

pituitary gland

parathyroid gland

thyroid gland

thymus gland

pancreas

adrenal glands

ovaries

RESPIRATORY SYSTEM

One thing in life that we have no choice in doing is breathing in and out, which is the function of the respiratory system. As a result, oxygen helps release energy for metabolism (energy comes mainly from sugar). Conversely, waste carbon dioxide passes from the cells into the bloodstream and is expelled.

The principal parts of this system are:

- **The trachea (windpipe)**, which leads into a system of branching tubes (the **bronchi** and **bronchiole**), through which air passes to and from the lungs.
- **The diaphragm**, which, when relaxed, is a dome-shaped sheet of muscle separating the chest cavity from the abdomen. When it contracts and flattens, it enlarges the chest cavity, expanding and drawing air into the lungs. When the **rib muscles** contract, it relaxes and air is forced out of the lungs.
- **The lungs**, which contain tiny air sacs called **alveoli**, richly supplied with blood capillaries. On breathing in, oxygen passes from the air into the blood. On breathing out, carbon dioxide passes from the blood into the air.

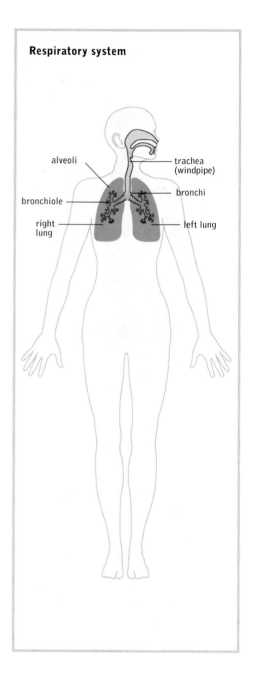

Respiratory system

- alveoli
- trachea (windpipe)
- bronchi
- bronchiole
- right lung
- left lung

Sinuses

These are air-filled spaces lined with mucous membranes that lie within the bone around the eyes and nose. If you get a cold, your nose and eyes become congested as the sinus cavity fills with mucus. Reflexology on the hands is a great way to drain the sinuses (see page 62).

DIGESTIVE SYSTEM

Digestion begins when food enters the mouth and ends when it is expelled as waste. The movement of food through the system is called **peristalsis**. The function of the digestive system is to process the carbohydrates, proteins and fats contained in food before the body can absorb them.

The main areas of activity are:

- **The mouth,** where the chewing action of the teeth and enzyme action breaks down the food into smaller particles, ready for further digestion.
- **The stomach,** where acid is secreted onto the food particles, enabling the stomach enzymes to break them down still further.
- **The small intestine,** where a combination of alkaline substances from the gall bladder and enzymes and juices from the pancreas complete the digestion of food. It is here that absorption of nutrients takes place.
- **The large intestine,** where water is absorbed from indigestible substances before they are passed out of the body as faeces.

Liver

This is the largest organ in the body, lying between the blood vessels carrying blood from the gut and those carrying blood to the heart, a prime position for filtering toxins from the blood. The gall bladder lies below it.

Pancreas

There are two types of cells in this gland. One produces pancreatic juice which flows through ducts into the small intestine. The other produces the hormone insulin which passes directly into the blood.

Digestive system

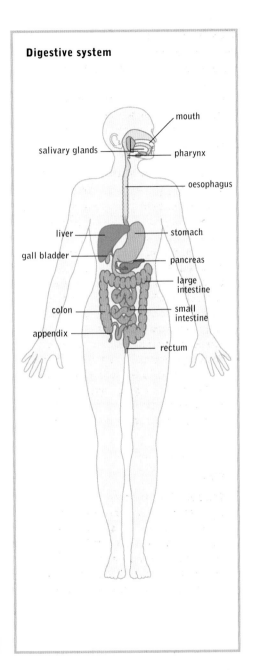

- mouth
- salivary glands
- pharynx
- oesophagus
- liver
- stomach
- gall bladder
- pancreas
- large intestine
- colon
- small intestine
- appendix
- rectum

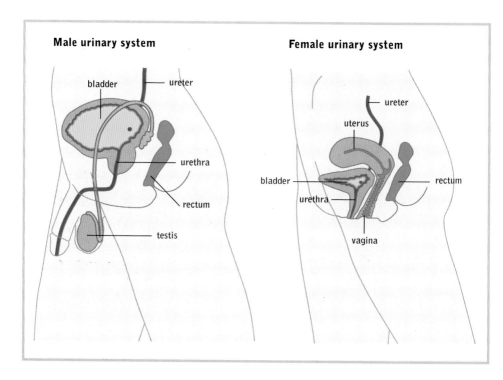

Male urinary system

- bladder
- ureter
- urethra
- rectum
- testis

Female urinary system

- ureter
- uterus
- bladder
- rectum
- urethra
- vagina

URINARY (EXCRETORY) SYSTEM

The urinary system is responsible for excreting waste substances and controlling the amount of water in the body: too much and water is dammed up in the tissues; too little and we become dehydrated.

The principal parts are:

- **The kidneys**, which are paired, bean-shaped structures in the lower back. Each consists of a collection of tubules that extract waste substances and excess water from the blood. This passes out of the body as **urine**.
- **The ureter**, which carries the urine from the kidneys to the bladder.
- **The bladder**, a bag of muscle where urine accumulates.
- **The urethra**, through which the urine is discharged from the body. In the female, this is short and quite separate from the opening of the reproductive system (the vagina). It is much longer in the male and carries sperm as well as urine out through the penis.

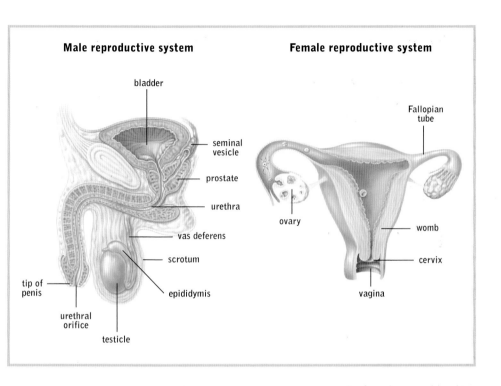

Male reproductive system

- bladder
- seminal vesicle
- prostate
- urethra
- vas deferens
- scrotum
- tip of penis
- epididymis
- urethral orifice
- testicle

Female reproductive system

- Fallopian tube
- ovary
- womb
- cervix
- vagina

REPRODUCTIVE SYSTEMS

This is closely linked with the urinary system, especially in the male.

The main organs in the male are:

- **The testicles**, which are stimulated into action by secretions of the pituitary gland, to produce sperm.
- **The sperm ducts (vas deferens)**, which carry the sperm to the urethra.
- **The prostate gland**, which provides lubrication for the sperm.
- **The urethra**, which passes through the penis.

The main organs in the female are:

- **The ovaries**, which are stimulated by pituitary gland secretions. They produce an egg about every 28 days and also secrete hormones.
- **The oviducts (Fallopian tubes)**, which carry the eggs to the womb.
- **The womb (uterus)**, which, stimulated by hormones from the ovaries, prepares to receive the egg by producing a blood-enriched lining. If an egg is fertilized by a sperm, it will embed itself into the lining and begin to develop into a baby, so that the woman becomes **pregnant**. If the egg is not fertilized, the lining of the womb is discarded and passes out of the body through the **vagina**. This discharge is known as a period, or menstruation.

Once beyond child-bearing age, a woman produces no more eggs and her periods stop. This marks the onset of the **menopause**.

ANATOMY OF THE HAND

In reflexology, it is important to have a basic understanding of the structure of the hand in order to better appreciate the location of reflexes and their stimulation.

BONES AND JOINTS

The hand contains 27 bones, which are held together with ligaments, tendons and muscles. There are three types:

1 **Wrist bones, or carpals** – there are eight in each wrist.
2 **Hand bones, or metacarpals** – there are five in each hand.
3 **Finger bones, or phalanges** – there are three in each finger and two in the thumb.

In addition, there are three types of joint:

1 **The hinge joints**, which are found in the finger bones and whose action resembles that of a door in that they 'open and shut' in one plane only.
2 **The gliding joints**, between the wrist bones, which allow less freedom of movement. Small fluid-filled sacs, or bursa, between the joints allow the bones to move over each other easily.
3 **The saddle joint**, which is unique and found only in the thumb.

Ossification

This is the process whereby different joints fuse at different stages of childhood. In babies, the top of the skull remains soft until the sutures fuse together at the age of about one year. The wrist bones in a newborn baby are not fused either, but, by the time he/she is 11 years old, the spaces between the joints will have grown smaller. When the joints have fused they are known as **fixed joints**.

FINGERNAILS AND SKIN

The fingertips contain a nail plate, which is attached to a matrix containing a delicate mesh of tiny capillaries. Any damage to the nail plate affects the growth and appearance of the nail. Both nails and skin are made of a horny substance called **keratin**. The skin on the palm of the hand (and on the sole of the foot) is unlike that of the rest of the body, and contains no hair follicles or sebaceous glands.

BLOOD AND NERVE SUPPLY

The hand is richly supplied with blood vessels. Indeed, they form such a dense conglomeration that it is easy to see why congestion occurs. This can be cleared with manual pressure during a reflexology session. There are also countless nerve endings in the hand, particularly in the fingertips, which is why they are so sensitive.

THE AGEING HAND

With age, the hand becomes more delicate, due to conditions such as osteoporosis (loss of bone density) or arthritis. Therefore, when treating a person, it is important to work gently over the reflexes, taking special care over delicate areas, such as prominent blood vessels or where the skin is thin.

Bones and joints of the hands

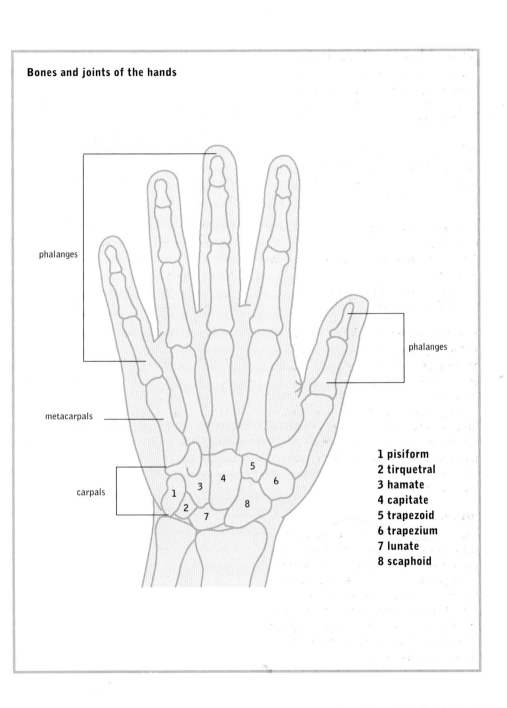

phalanges

phalanges

metacarpals

carpals

1 pisiform
2 tirquetral
3 hamate
4 capitate
5 trapezoid
6 trapezium
7 lunate
8 scaphoid

a hand reflexology session

Before starting any reflexology session, you should prepare both yourself and the location where the session is to take place. If you are treating a partner, it is important to consider any hand conditions that he/she may be experiencing and adapt your treatment accordingly.

Every session should open and close with a set series of moves and you should be familiar with the basic techniques involved. There are six basic moves, all of which are fully described and illustrated. However, you should always feel free to improvise.

things to bear in mind

Before starting any reflexology session, there are some things to take into consideration.

THE HOLISTIC APPROACH TO HEALTH

The word 'holistic' derives from *holos*, meaning 'whole' in Greek. Like most integrative therapies, reflexology uses this approach, which has a very positive effect on health. You should always view a condition in the context of the whole body; for example, a pain in the shoulder may be due to a back problem. This means considering all the factors that are currently affecting a person.

Harmony between the body, mind and spirit is essential as no single element can work alone. There are three major considerations:

1 The physical body – the organs and structures which are out of balance within their environment.
2 The emotional body (mind) – how people feel within themselves and their everyday reactions to stress and interaction with others.
3 The energy body (spirit) – this can only be explained by saying that every single cell in the human body has an electrical charge, which is a form of energy.

CONTRAINDICATIONS

It is most important to look at and assess the hand before starting any treatment. Use your common sense and instincts – it is advisable not to treat anyone with a contagious disease, such as chickenpox, because of the risk of passing it on to someone else. **Contraindications** include:

- Rheumatoid arthritis and other forms of arthritis resulting from inflammation in the space between the joints – treatment can cause physical pain and damage, so be sensitive and careful, paying attention to reactions.
- Cuts, sprains, blisters, scabs, rashes, whitlows, infections and fissures.
- Chilblains, Raynaud's disorders and very cold hands – spend more preparation time on opening and closing movements.
- Delicate hands, as in the very old and the very young.
- Diseases of the nervous system (mainly Parkinson's and delirium tremors from alcohol abuse) – use a firm grip, but a light pressure and gentle treatment process.
- Swollen areas which are painful to touch – you may find it useful to treat above or below the site of pain.
- Mental health conditions – it is important to set up boundaries when treating someone with a mental problem, even if it is a member of your family or a friend.

ADAPTING TREATMENT

In some cases you may need to adapt your normal hand reflexology session.

- **Young children** – use a lighter pressure and a shorter treatment time. A parent or guardian should be present. Provide toys to create an informal relaxed atmosphere and allow extra time to establish a rapport.
- **The frail and elderly** – use a lighter pressure with a slow rhythm and do not place undue emphasis on specific reflexes. Use more relaxation techniques and generally a shorter treatment time, but leave some time for talking.
- **People with terminal illness** – give a lighter treatment with more emphasis on pain relief. Treatments should be shorter but more frequent, with more time for relaxation and reassurance.

- **Nervous subjects** – reassure them that the treatment is not painful and mention its benefits. Demonstrate on the hand before starting treatment.
- **Pregnant women** – place more emphasis on the spine and lymphatic work.
- **Injured people** – use cross-reflexes (see page 24) to avoid the site of injury.

REACTIONS TO TREATMENT

Initially the body may respond to treatment by severe but temporary worsening of symptoms or by the appearance of apparently new acute symptoms. This is known as a **healing crisis** and should be followed by an improvement in the condition. It may be seen as a turning point in the illness and is a positive occurrence, indicating that the body is responding to treatment.

The following reactions to a reflexology treatment are quite common:

- Temporary worsening of symptoms.
- Runny nose or cold-like symptoms.
- Headache.
- Skin reaction, especially on the hand – the skin is expelling toxins.
- Increased sweating, especially from the hands and feet.
- Increased thirst – drinking aids the process of ridding toxins.
- Increased urination and more frequent bowel movements.
- Feeling cold or hot – if cold, the blood is feeding internal organs; if hot, it is feeding the more outer-lying part of the body, such as muscles and skin.
- Feeling emotional, to the point of crying, or being 'on a high'.
- Feeling tired or full of energy – the result of improved circulation.

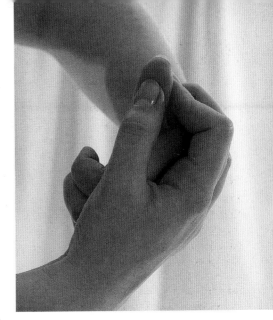

Above: During a treatment you may feel different sensations in your hand. Generally the sensations should be pleasant and soothing, but congested reflexes may be more sensitive.

- Feeling irritable or restless, or deeply relaxed.
- Increased movement in the hands – the result of manipulation during reflexology.
- Sounder sleep.
- Disappearance of symptoms or relief of pain.

We react to treatments in this way because:

- It is part of the **healing process**.
- There is a release of toxins into the body – working on the reflex points breaks up the lactic acid and calcium crystals which have built up around the nerve endings in the feet or hands (7,200 in the hands, but fewer in the feet).
- Rebalancing energy pathways releases tension or pent-up emotions.

After a treatment has come to an end, it is important to **drink plenty of water** to help flush toxins from the system.

preparation

Thorough preparation and a professional approach to hand reflexology will give both you and your client confidence.

STEP 1: PREPARING YOURSELF

When treating others, it is important to present yourself professionally, and the first step is to prepare yourself.

- Make sure your hands are in good condition and your nails are short.
- Remove all jewellery and your watch.

STEP 2: SETTING THE SCENE

You should 'set the scene' before commencing any reflexology treatment, whether on yourself or on somebody else. This is known as **healing space**. You should provide:

- A quiet place free from telephones or other disturbances.
- Comfortable seating.
- Fresh air.
- A glass of water.
- A clean pillow or towel on which to place the subject's hands and a towel with which to cover them.

STEP 3: SITTING COMFORTABLY

It is very important that both you and the subject feel comfortable during a hand reflexology session and that you have easy access to their hands. Be sure to establish eye contact with your subject and ask them to remove all of their jewellery and their watch. There are six different positions (see right) that you can try when giving a reflexology treatment – but there is always scope for improvisation.

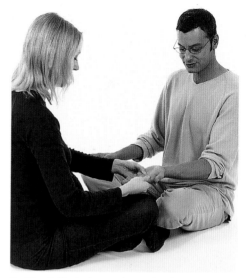

Position 1 Seated opposite each other.

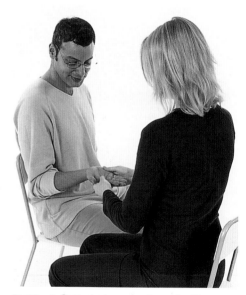

Position 2 Seated criss-cross to each other.

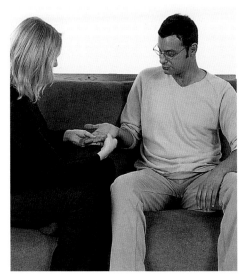

Position 3 Seated close on a sofa.

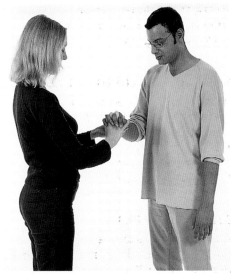

Position 5 Standing opposite each other.

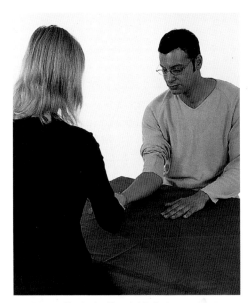

Position 4 Seated with a table between you.

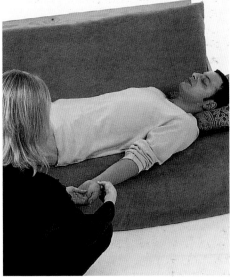

Position 6 With the subject lying down and the therapist sitting alongside.

STEP 4: CHECKING FOR CONTRAINDICATIONS

Check for any hand conditions (see page 42) that may stop you going ahead with a treatment or make you treat more carefully than normal. You should also check the hand for cuts, bruises, etc. Hold the subject's hands in yours for a moment before you start. It does not matter how you hold them, just do what feels natural.

STEP 5: POSITIONING THE HAND

The hand is best placed on a pillow, although this is not essential providing that both you and your subject are comfortable. Place a towel over any area that has been treated. Once you have completed work on one hand, cover it with a towel.

STEP 6: SETTING A GOAL

Decide what you want to achieve; for example, are you treating for:

• Stress relief?
• Detoxification?
• Pain relief?
• Improved circulation?

STEP 7: TIMING

Allow about 10–20 minutes to conduct a complete session on both hands.

STEP 8: PRESSURE

This should range from light to hard (one to three). You can use more pressure on the palm of the hand than on the back, where there are more blood vessels, tendons and ligaments and it can be painful if worked too hard. Work within your subject's pain threshold; communication and

developing a rapport are important, so watch the facial expression when exerting pressure. It is essential to pay careful attention to sensitive areas: work them slowly at first using skin tension, as often the reflexes are deeply buried. Then increase the pressure within the boundaries of the client's threshold of pain.

Will the treatment hurt?

Treatment is usually pleasant, but some reflex points may be tender. However, any pain should only last briefly. Some causes of pain are:

• Injury or a scar from a past injury.
• Conditions requiring surgery, both before and after the operation.
• Stress and anxiety – which may cause oversensitivity.
• Drugs and medication – prescription drugs may oversensitize or numb the reflexes.
• Illness – which may make the reflexes very sensitive if the subject's condition is in an acute phase.

How many treatments and how often?

The number and frequency of treatments depends on your needs and those of your subject. Each person is different and everyone responds differently to treatment. It may be useful to take notes following each session. After the first six treatments, any improvement should be evident, so this is a good point at which to review the situation. You may need to take into account the seriousness of the condition and how long the subject has been living with it.

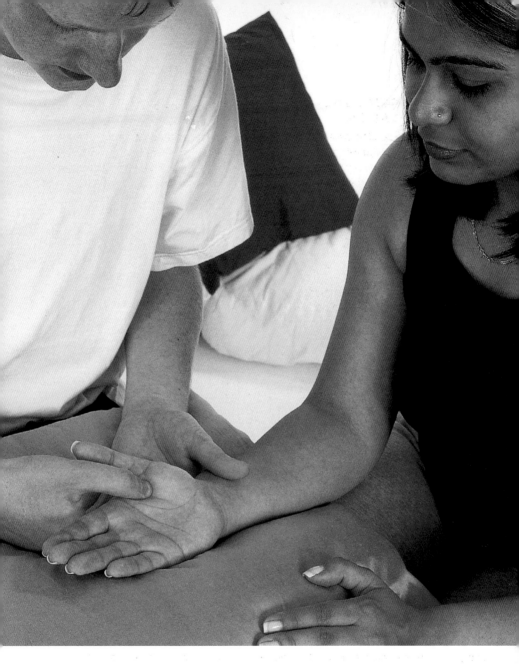

Above: *Check the medical history (past and present) of your partner to help your approach to their treatment. If there is any doubt about a condition or injury, ask your partner to refer to their doctor for advice.*

opening moves

Every reflexology session should begin with this series of movements, which you can also use on yourself. Note that you should always begin any treatment with the **right** hand.

Before embarking on any reflexology treatment, you need to open the hand in order to relax both the structure and the person being treated. Begin with five minutes of relaxation movements. You can repeat these several times until you feel comfortable to go on or the person feels ready. There are **three** opening movements.

1 WRIST ROTATION

Clasp your partner's hand in yours, palm to palm, interlocking fingers, and use your other hand to support the wrist. Now rotate the hand in each direction to loosen the wrist structure.

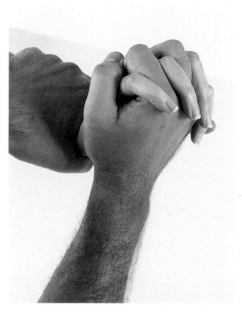

2 FINGER PULL

Clasp your partner's hand as before. Pull the interlocked fingers out very slowly as you exert pressure at the tips.

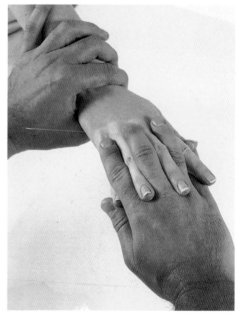

3 WRIST PUSH AND PULL

Clasp your partner's hand as before. Push the hand back for five seconds (left), then pull it forward for five seconds (bottom left).

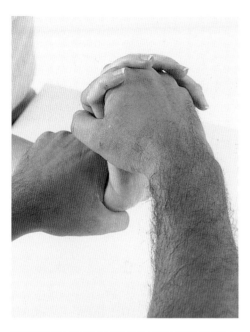

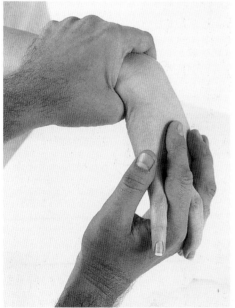

Taking care of your hands

Touch is an important part of reflexology, so take care of your hands – you only have one pair!

- Soak your hands in warm olive oil with a stimulant such as menthol or peppermint oil.
- Cut your nails short regularly and moisturize your hands daily.

closing moves

There are **four** movements which should be used at the close of any hand reflexology session. Like the opening movements, you can use these on yourself. Just improvise and imagine that you are treating someone else's hands.

1 FINGER ROTATION

Support your partner's wrist with one hand and use the other hand to support and rotate each finger separately. This energizing move closes the hand and clears each zone of energy.

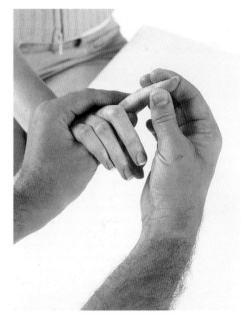

2 FIST ROLL

Form a fist with one of your hands, place your partner's palm on the knuckles of your hand, then place your other hand palm down on the dorsal aspect of their hand and rotate it; this is calming and relaxing. To treat yourself, place the fist into the palm of your other hand, then roll, to work the dorsal and palmar aspects.

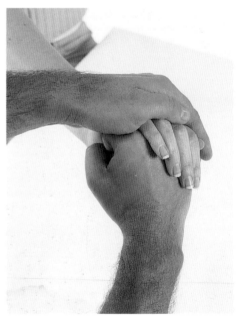

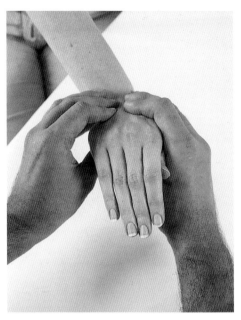

3 WRIST DRAINAGE

Support your partner's hand by placing your thumbs under their lower palm and your fingers dorsally on their wrist. Then use your fingers to drain the hand, up the lymphatic reflex, along the wrist and forearm.

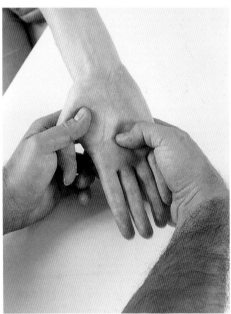

4 SOLAR PLEXUS

Place your partner's hand palm upward and place your thumb in the centre of their palm. As you exert pressure using the tornado (see page 55), ask your partner to breathe deeply and to hold his/her breath for three seconds; release the pressure as he/she releases the breath. Repeat three times. Now turn over your partner's hand and place your palms directly above, but not touching, their dorsal aspect. With your eyes closed (and your partner's), transfer healing thoughts as you imagine taking away his/her negative energy.

basic techniques

There are **six** basic moves, but feel free to improvise or to elaborate on each of them. Some moves work together to become another move – this is known as morphing; for example, the butterfly progresses into the caterpillar, and tearing progresses into the tornado. Each of these moves can be used either on yourself or someone else.

 BUTTERFLY

 CATERPILLAR

 HOOKING

 BIRD'S BEAK

 TEARING

 TORNADO

1 BUTTERFLY

First practise the finger position; look at the medial side of the hand and bend the index finger so both finger joints are closed. Place the thumb of the same hand on the finger joint so that the tip over-rides the index finger joint and the thumb can move up and down, with the index finger as a supporting bridge. Practise by applying the butterfly to an area of the hand, depressing and raising the thumbtip over a reflex area. The butterfly is used to criss-cross the **diaphragm** reflex and can also become a caterpillar, as in the areas of the **teeth** and **jaw** reflexes.

Self

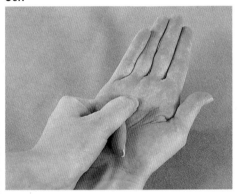

With partner

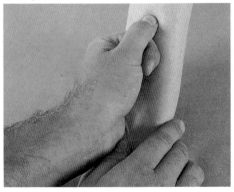

2 CATERPILLAR

This move is just as it sounds. Move your thumb or index finger in caterpillar fashion, unlocking and relocking each finger joint as you exert pressure along the zone. It is important to establish some skin tension around the area that you caterpillar over. This is an alternating pressure technique, in which the tip of the thumb presses down, lifts up and presses down again in tiny bites. Imagine a caterpillar walking along a leaf and, when you hit a reflex point, eating the leaf. Establish a moderate rhythm. The caterpillar is used on the reflexes of the **head, neck** and **sinuses.**

Self

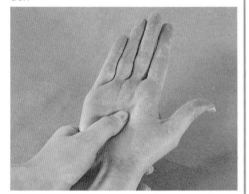

With partner

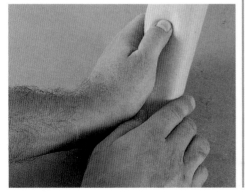

3 HOOKING

Form a 'hook' by bending the thumb, the thumbtip being the end of the hook. Use this hook to gouge into a specific reflex point, then work the area until any deposits are destroyed or any pain subsides. The idea is to hook in and push up and down medially or laterally, imagining that the specific reflex point is hidden and must be located and stimulated. Hooking is used for the **occipital** reflex and, on the right hand, for the **pancreas** reflex.

Self

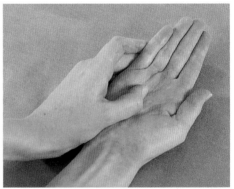

With partner

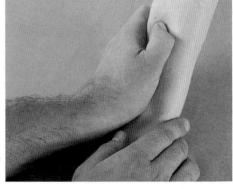

4 BIRD'S BEAK

Press the tip of your thumb against your fingertip to form a 'beak'; this action involves forming the beginning of a pinch, but not actually pinching. Go to the area of the hand that you want to cross and, keeping the tip of your thumb pressed against your finger, begin walking the tip of the index finger, leaving the thumb behind. Continue over the area, becoming a caterpillar – morphing from a move transcends your technique to another level! The bird's beak is used on the **lymphatics** reflex between the fingers on the dorsal aspect of the hand, among others.

Self

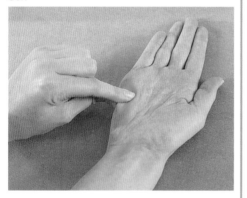

With partner

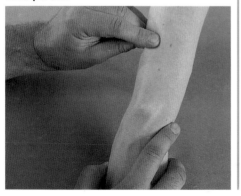

5 TEARING

This move is like the caterpillar, but in order to get to the more hidden or tough, resistant reflexes you have to really tear, usually laterally, to hit the reflex point; the firmer you tear, the greater the stimulation. This is where the therapeutic aspect begins, because the reflex point is stimulated by the tearing motion. The move is more about what you are trying to tear – a very thick material – although it never gets truly torn. Tearing is ideal for the **knee** and **hip** reflexes.

Self

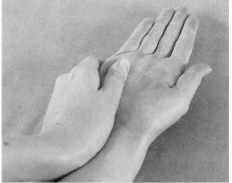

With partner

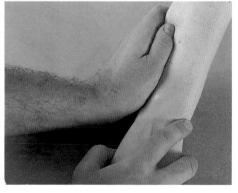

6 TORNADO

This move is as simple as it sounds. Point your thumb directly downwards as if drilling a hole and rotate it clockwise and anticlockwise continuously as you either break down the deposits or the reflex gets less painful. This move is particularly suited for the **pituitary** reflex, where the continuous rotation penetrates the reflexology point.

Underlying causes

It is important to remember that many common conditions – for example, irritable bowel syndrome, tension headaches and insomnia – are compounded by stress, which may be an underlying cause. Relieving stress with effective hand reflexology techniques will relax and balance the body's systems and have a positive effect on the manifested symptoms.

Self

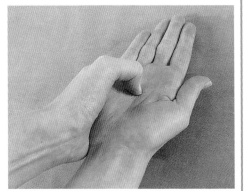

With partner

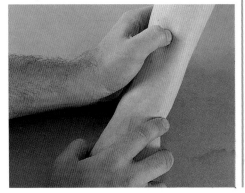

Strengthening exercises for your hands

If you intend to do a lot of reflexology, it is helpful to practise a few simple exercises to strengthen your hands and arms.

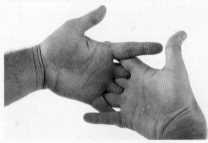

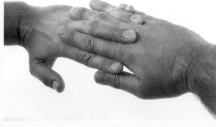

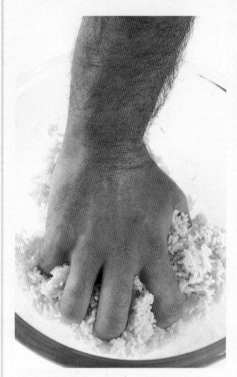

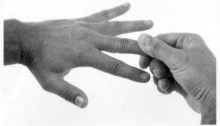

- Boil some rice until it is overcooked, leave it in a bowl to cool, then add some paprika or cayenne pepper (to stimulate the blood supply to your skin). Put both hands into the bowl, take a handful of rice in each hand and squeeze it. Repeat this for about 10 minutes. This will work and strengthen the smaller muscles of the hands.

- Clasp your fingers and pull your hands away from each other. Next, pull each finger in turn.

how to use the treatments

The following chapters give simple but effective hand reflexology treatments that are **easy to apply** and **easy to remember** – find the relevant sequence to help with your own or your partner's particular condition and use the moves each day to relieve the symptoms. The techniques can be practised on a bus or train on the way to or back from the office, or as a quick fix any time during the day, since no special equipment is required and the movements are small, inconspicuous and unobtrusive.

When carrying out a treatment, follow the sequence instructions and position of the reflex points carefully, keeping in mind the timings, the amount of pressure that should be applied and the instruction symbol for each movement. It is essential to meet the needs of the person who is having the treatment and that includes yourself, so it is important not to apply any more pressure than is needed. A hand reflexology treatment should be **a pleasurable experience**, so the object is not to feel pain.

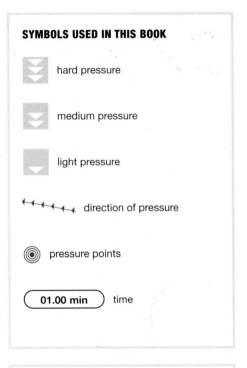

SYMBOLS USED IN THIS BOOK

hard pressure

medium pressure

light pressure

direction of pressure

pressure points

01.00 min   time

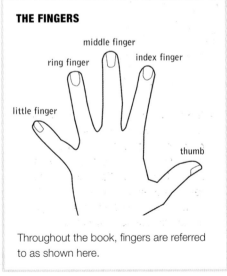

THE FINGERS

middle finger

ring finger

index finger

little finger

thumb

Throughout the book, fingers are referred to as shown here.

treating common conditions

Treating yourself: 10-minute treatments

There are a number of common conditions that affect most people at some time in their lives and for which reflexology provides a means of relief. In this chapter, these conditions are grouped according to the parts or systems of the body, starting with the head and working down to the pelvis.

For each group of conditions, a hand reflexology sequence has been devised, which will take five minutes for each hand. Find somewhere comfortable to sit, relax and use the simple-to-follow steps to help relieve pain and tension in the related body areas.

head conditions

headache Pain felt all over the head or occuring in just one area. It may be superficial or deep, throbbing or sharp.

migraine A severe headache lasting from two hours to two days, preceded and accompanied by visual disturbances and/or nausea and vomiting.

eyestrain Aching or discomfort in or around the eyes, commonly associated with headaches, sinusitis, conjunctivitis, hay fever and inflammation of the eyelids.

conjunctivitis Inflammation of the conjunctiva of the eye causing redness, discomfort and a discharge from the affected area.

toothache Pain coming from one or more teeth or from the gums, felt as a dull throb or as a sharp twinge.

To help with these conditions, work on the following reflexes:

Head

Neck

Eye

Teeth

Kidney/Adrenal glands

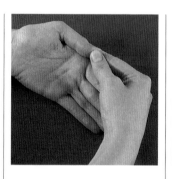

1 Head reflex

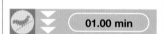

01.00 min

Cup one thumb in your other hand. Use your working thumb to walk down from the tip to the base of the thumb. Continue in this manner until you have covered the area. Stimulate with tiny circles at each step.

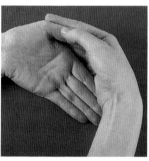

2 Neck reflex

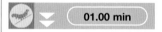

01.00 min

Cup one thumb in the other hand so that it is resting between your index and middle fingers. Use your working thumb to walk along the bone of the thumb from the first to the second joint. Make seven small steps along the bone, to represent the seven vertebrae in the neck.

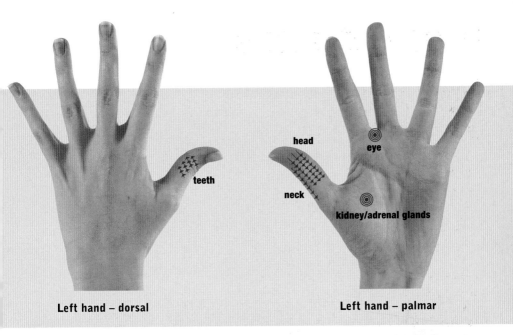

head

eye

teeth

neck

kidney/adrenal glands

Left hand – dorsal

Left hand – palmar

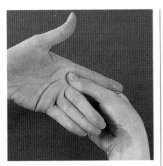

3 Eye reflex

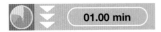

`01.00 min`

Support one hand in your other hand. Place your working thumb between the index and middle fingers, apply pressure and tear towards the joint at the base of the second finger. Stimulate with small circles.

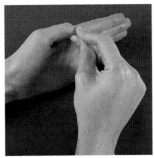

4 Teeth reflex

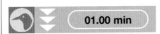

`01.00 min`

Support your thumb. Use your working index finger and thumb to walk between your thumbnail and the first joint.

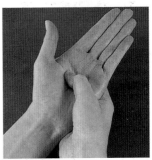

5 Kidney/Adrenal glands reflex

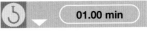

`01.00 min`

Support one hand in the other. Place your working thumb in the webbing between the thumb and index finger just above the thumb muscle halfway down the hand. Use your thumb to hook into the webbing and apply an even pressure.

treating common conditions 61

ear, nose and throat conditions

sinusitis Inflammation of the membrane lining the facial sinuses. Accompanied by tension or a throbbing ache and may cause fever, a stuffy nose and a loss of the sense of smell.

dizziness Light-headedness, unsteadiness or sense of surroundings spinning. Caused by stress, tiredness, fever or a sudden drop of blood flow to the brain.

rhinitis Inflammation of the nasal membranes, often from an allergy, leading to nasal congestion and an increase in mucus production.

tinnitus Ringing, humming, buzzing, whistling or other, usually constant, noise in the ear, which is not caused by external noise. It can worsen with stress.

hearing loss Most commonly caused by ageing. It can also result from damage or infection to any part of the outer, middle or inner ear.

To help with these conditions, work on the following reflexes:

Sinuses

Eustachian tube

Outer ear

Inner ear

Kidney/Adrenal glands

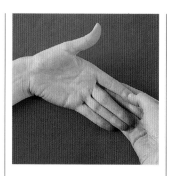

1 Sinuses reflex

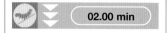
02.00 min

Support the fingers of one hand in the other. Using your working thumb, walk from the tip to the base, or the base to the tip, of the index finger. Continue in this manner until you have worked all the fingers. Stimulate with tiny circles at each step.

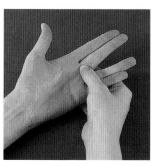

2 Eustachian tube reflex

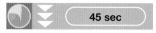
45 sec

Support one hand in the other. Place your working thumb between the middle and ring fingers. Apply pressure, tear towards the joint at the base of the middle finger and stimulate with small circles.

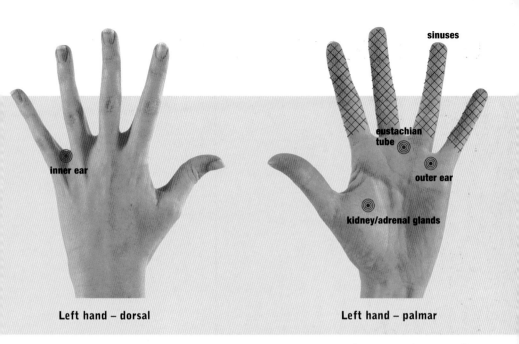

sinuses

eustachian
tube

inner ear

outer ear

kidney/adrenal glands

Left hand – dorsal

Left hand – palmar

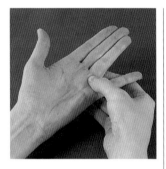

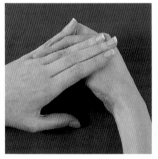

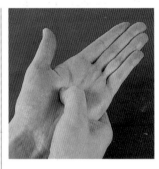

3 Outer ear reflex

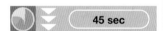 45 sec

Support one hand in the other.
Place your working thumb
between the ring and little
fingers. Apply pressure, tear
towards the joint at the base of
the little finger and stimulate
with small circles.

4 Inner ear reflex

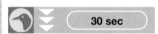 30 sec

Place your hand palm downward.
Place your working index finger
and thumb on the joint at the
base of the ring finger. Apply
pressure and make small circles
to stimulate.

**5 Kidney/Adrenal
glands reflex**

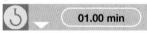 01.00 min

Support one hand in the other.
Place your working thumb in
the webbing between the thumb
and index finger just above the
thumb muscle halfway down the
hand. Use your thumb to hook
into the webbing and apply an
even pressure.

neck and shoulder conditions

neck pain Can be caused by tension, arthritis in the neck bones, swollen glands, referred pain, compression of the nerves in the neck or injury.

whiplash Injury to the soft tissues and spinal joints of the neck, from sudden violent forward then backward movement. Symptoms are usually worse after 24 hours.

cervical spondylosis (cervical osteoarthritis) Degenerative disorder affecting the joints between the neck bones and causing pain and stiffness in the neck.

bursitis (shoulder) Usually the result of pressure, friction or slight injury to the bursa (fluid-filled sac) surrounding the shoulder joint.

frozen shoulder Stiffness and pain caused by inflammation of the lining of the capsule surrounding the shoulder joint. Normal movement is difficult, even impossible.

To help with these conditions, work on the following reflexes:

Neck

Shoulder

Occipital bone

Upper spine

Kidney/Adrenal glands

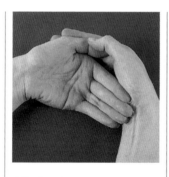

1 Neck reflex

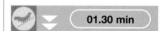 01.30 min

Cup one thumb in the other hand so that it is resting between your index and middle fingers. Use your working thumb to walk along the bone of the thumb from the first to the second joint. Make seven small steps along the bone, to represent the seven vertebrae in the neck.

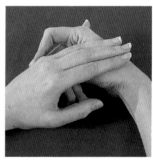

2 Shoulder reflex

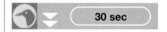 30 sec

Place one hand palm downward. Place your working index finger and thumb between the base of the ring and little fingers. Apply pressure and, using bird's beak, take three tiny steps towards the wrist and stimulate the area with small circles.

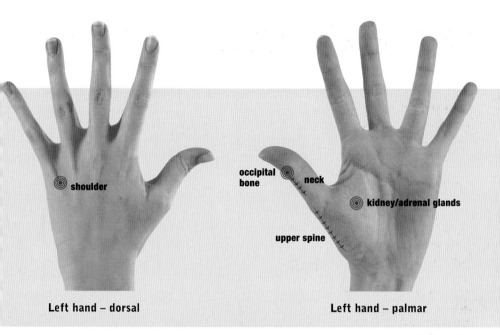

shoulder

occipital bone

neck

kidney/adrenal glands

upper spine

Left hand – dorsal

Left hand – palmar

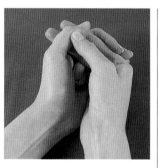

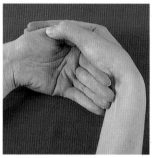

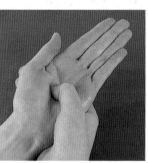

3 Occipital bone reflex

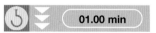 01.00 min

Place your working thumb against the first joint of the other thumb. Hook up against the bone and stimulate in clockwise or anticlockwise circles.

4 Upper spine reflex

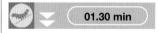 01.30 min

Cup one hand in the other, so that your working thumb rests on the bone at the base of the thumb. Make 12 small steps along the bone to the edge of the wrist, to represent the 12 vertebrae in the upper spine. Stimulate with small circles at each step.

5 Kidney/Adrenal glands reflex

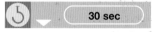 30 sec

Support one hand in the other. Place your working thumb in the webbing between the thumb and index finger just above the thumb muscle halfway down the hand. Use your thumb to hook into the webbing and apply an even pressure.

hand and wrist conditions

tenosynovitis Inflammation of the inner lining of the sheath that surrounds a tendon (commonly those of the hand and the wrist), often caused by overuse.

carpal tunnel syndrome Pain, numbness, and pins and needles in the thumb, index and middle fingers of one or both hands. Grip may be weak.

repetitive strain injury (rsi) Overuse of the finger and the wrist joints causing symptoms of pain and stiffness in the affected joints.

tennis elbow Pain and tenderness on the back of the forearm and the outside of the elbow, usually from overuse of the muscles.

raynaud's disease Restriction of blood flow to the fingers, which can lead to white, numb areas. There may be considerable pain, numbness or tingling.

To help with these conditions, work on the following reflexes:

Wrist

Elbow

Shoulder

Neck

Kidney/Adrenal glands

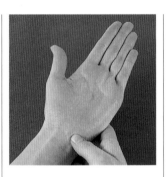

1 Wrist reflex

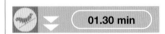 01.30 min

Place your working thumb at one side of the wrist and caterpillar walk at the base of the hand from one side of the wrist to the other. Stimulate with small circles at each step. Repeat.

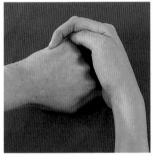

2 Elbow reflex

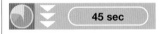 45 sec

Place one hand palm downward. Place your working index finger at the side of the hand just at the base of the little finger. Make two tiny steps towards the wrist with your index finger and tear back towards the fingers.

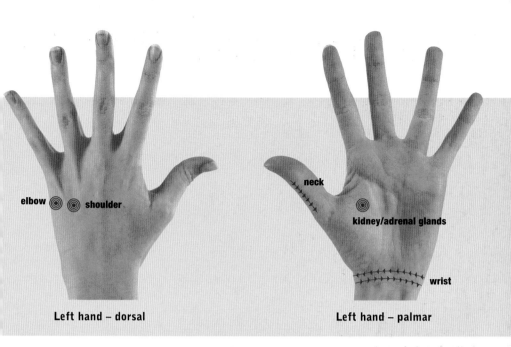

elbow ⊚ ⊚ shoulder

neck

kidney/adrenal glands

wrist

Left hand – dorsal

Left hand – palmar

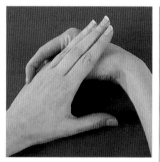

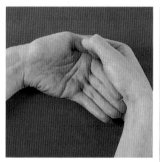

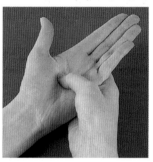

3 Shoulder reflex

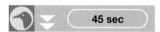 45 sec

Place one hand palm downward. Place your working index finger and thumb between the bases of the ring and little fingers. Apply pressure, then bird's beak three tiny steps towards the wrist and stimulate with small circles.

4 Neck reflex

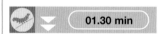 01.30 min

Cup one thumb in the other hand so that it is resting between your index and middle fingers. Use your working thumb to walk along the bone of the thumb from the first to the second joint. Make seven small steps along the bone, to represent the seven vertebrae in the neck.

5 Kidney/Adrenals glands reflex

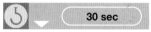 30 sec

Support one hand in the other. Place your working thumb in the webbing between the thumb and index finger just above the thumb muscle halfway down the hand. Use your thumb to hook into the webbing and apply pressure.

respiratory conditions

asthma An allergic condition affecting the lungs that results in breathing difficulties such as wheezing, sweating, increased heartbeat and coughing as the airways narrow.

common colds Infections of the upper respiratory tract, caused by numerous different viruses. Duration is about eight days, but colds may lead to more serious infections.

bronchitis The tubes that lead to the lungs (bronchi) become inflamed or obstructed, leading to excess mucus, fever, coughing, sore throat and breathing difficulty.

influenza Commonly known as 'flu' and spread by coughing or sneezing. Symptoms can include aching head and body, tiredness and fever alternating with chills.

sore throat Pain and tenderness in the passages running from the back of the mouth and nose to the upper part of the gullet.

To help with these conditions, work on the following reflexes:

Head

Throat/Hiatus hernia

Lungs

Kidney/Adrenal glands

Lymphatics

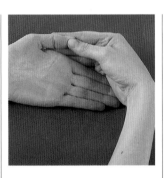

1 Head reflex

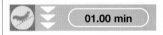 01.00 min

Cup one thumb in your other hand. Use your working thumb to walk down from the tip to the base of the thumb. Continue in this manner until you have covered the area. Stimulate with tiny circles at each step.

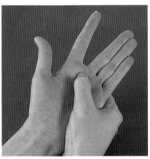

2 Throat/Hiatus hernia reflex

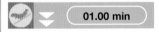 01.00 min

Place your working thumb on the hiatus hernia point and walk up between the bones to the bases of the index and the middle fingers. Continue in this manner, stimulating with small circles at each step.

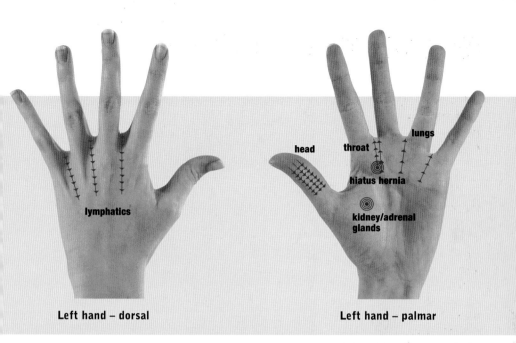

head **throat** **lungs**

hiatus hernia

lymphatics

kidney/adrenal glands

Left hand – dorsal   Left hand – palmar

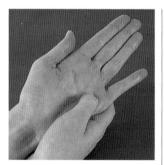

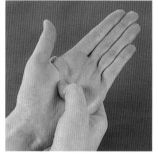

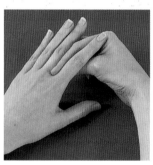

3 Lungs reflex

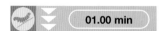 (01.00 min)

Place your working thumb halfway down the palm of the hand between zones 5 and 4. Apply pressure and use the caterpillar walk towards the base of the fingers and between the bones. Continue in this manner between zones 4 and 3 and zones 3 and 2.

4 Kidney/Adrenal glands reflex

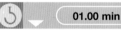 (01.00 min)

Support one hand in the other. Place your working thumb in the webbing between the thumb and index finger just above the thumb muscle halfway down the hand. Use your thumb to hook into the webbing and apply an even pressure.

5 Lymphatics reflex

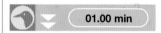 (01.00 min)

Place one hand palm downward. Place your working index finger and thumb between the bases of the index and middle fingers. Apply pressure and, using bird's beak, take tiny steps towards the wrist. Continue in this manner between zones 3 and 4 and zones 4 and 5.

digestive conditions

acid reflux Condition caused by acid liquid rising from the stomach into the oesophagus (the tube connecting the stomach and throat). Common symptoms include a sour taste in the mouth and burning sensations on eating.

heartburn A burning pain that travels up from the centre of the chest to the throat, often exacerbated by bending over or lying down.

nausea Feeling a need to vomit, which is often accompanied by paleness and excessive sweating.

indigestion The incomplete digestion of foods in the stomach or intestines. Symptoms include heartburn, nausea, bloating, passing wind, abdominal pain and a sensation of fullness.

hiatus hernia A weakness in the diaphragm that allows stomach contents to wash upward into the gullet. Symptoms include heartburn and acid reflux.

To help with these conditions, work on the following reflexes:

Stomach

Diaphragm

Hiatus hernia

Throat

Pancreas

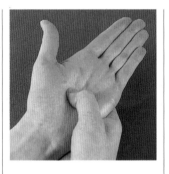

1 Stomach reflex

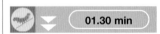 01.30 min

Support one hand in the other. Place your working thumb at the tip of the webbing between the thumb and index finger. Then walk to the edge of the hand and return back to your original point. Continue until you have covered the webbing, rather like the spokes of a bicycle wheel.

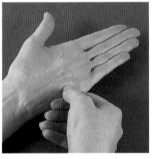

2 Diaphragm reflex

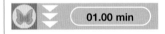 01.00 min

Place your working thumb a third of the way down the palm of your other hand. Use the butterfly movement to walk across the hand from one side to the other.

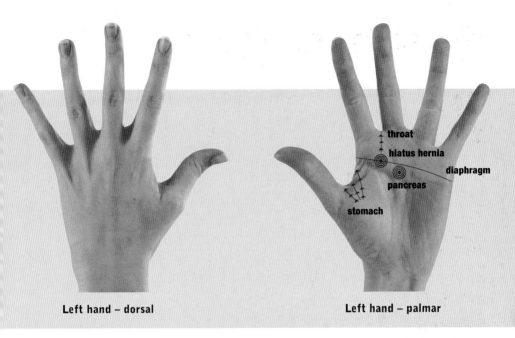

Left hand – dorsal

Left hand – palmar

throat
hiatus hernia
diaphragm
pancreas
stomach

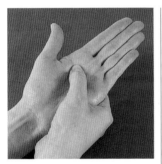

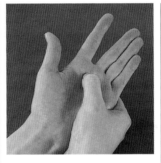

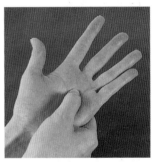

3 Hiatus hernia reflex

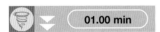 01.00 min

Place your working thumb on the diaphragm line between zones 2 and 3 and apply firm pressure.

4 Throat reflex

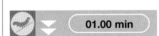 01.00 min

Place your working thumb on the hiatus hernia point and walk up between the bones to the bases of the index and middle fingers. Continue in this manner, stimulating with small circles at each step.

5 Pancreas reflex

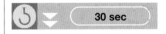 30 sec

Place your working thumb on the diaphragm line at the joint at the base of the middle finger. Hook up towards the ring finger and against the joint.

digestive conditions

food poisoning Commonly occurs after eating food containing harmful bacteria or toxins. Symptoms include vomiting, abdominal cramps, dizziness, diarrhoea, dehydration, nausea, chills, fever and a headache.

peptic ulcer Open wounds in the stomach lining or walls of the duodenum, caused by the acid of the stomach irritating the lining and the tissues beneath it.

constipation Occurs when waste material moves too slowly through the large bowel, resulting in hard, dry faeces and infrequent and painful bowel movements.

diarrhoea Frequent passing of unusually loose, watery stools and may be accompanied by vomiting, cramps, thirst and abdominal pain.

irritable bowel syndrome (ibs) Symptoms include irregular bowel movements, diarrhoea, constipation, bloating, abdominal pain, the accumulation of mucus in the stools, nausea and flatulence.

To help with these conditions, work on the following reflexes:

Stomach

Liver/Spleen

Large intestine

Small intestine

Autonomic nerves

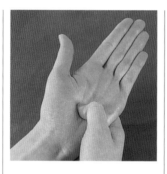

1 Stomach reflex

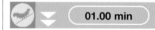 01.00 min

Support one hand in the other. Place your working thumb at the tip of the webbing between the thumb and index finger. Then walk to the edge of the hand and return back to your original point. Continue until you have covered the webbing, rather like the spokes of a bicycle wheel.

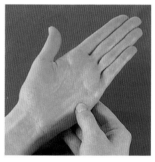

2 Liver (right hand)/Spleen (left hand) reflex

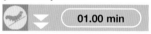 01.00 min

Place your working thumb on the edge of your other hand, one thumbprint down from the base of the little finger. Using the caterpillar walk, take three small steps into the hand. Continue in this manner for five lines, finishing just above the wrist.

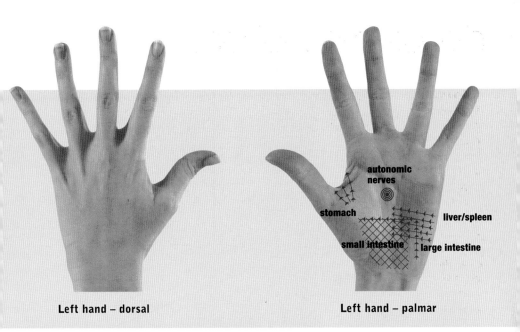

Left hand – dorsal

Left hand – palmar

(palmar labels) autonomic nerves · stomach · liver/spleen · small intestine · large intestine

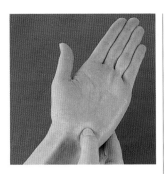

3 Large intestine reflex

01.00 min

Place your working thumb at the base of zone 4 just above the wrist. Turn your thumbnail so it faces up to the ring finger. Walk up zone 4 until halfway up the hand. Push down and stimulate before turning to walk across the hand, ending up between the webbing.

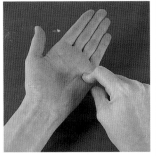

4 Small intestine reflex

01.00 min

Place your working index finger and thumb two fingerprints from the base of the fingers. Apply pressure and walk with tiny steps across the hand. Continue in this manner over the palm until you reach the wrist.

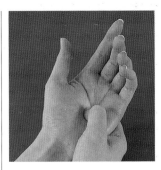

5 Autonomic nerves reflex

01.00 min

Place your working thumb in the centre of the palm. Relax your hand so that the fingers fall over the working thumb. Apply pressure and stimulate with small circles and take deep breaths.

urinary conditions

cystitis Inflammation of the lining of the bladder, usually caused by a bacterial infection. Main symptoms are a frequent urge to pass urine and pain.

incontinence More common in women, particularly after childbirth, this is the uncontrollable, involuntary passing of urine. Disease or injury of the urinary tract can also weaken bladder control.

bladder stones More common in men, these are hard build-ups of mineral located in the urinary bladder. Main symptoms are difficulty in passing urine and pain.

kidney stones These cause severe pain in the kidney area. More common in summer when urine becomes more concentrated due to fluid loss through sweat.

kidney infection Most often occurs as a result of bacteria ascending to the kidneys from the bladder. Symptoms can include backache, chills and fever.

To help with these conditions, work on the following reflexes:

Pituitary

Bladder

Ureter (Kidney tube)

Kidney/Adrenal glands

Lower back

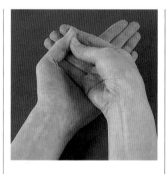

1 Pituitary reflex

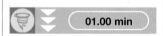
01.00 min

Support one thumb on the fingers of your other hand. Use your working thumb to apply pressure and stimulate the centre of your other thumb.

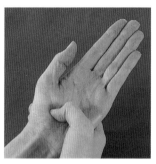

2 Bladder reflex

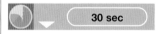
30 sec

Place your working thumb in the base of the muscle of the thumb. Tear down towards the wrist and stimulate this area.

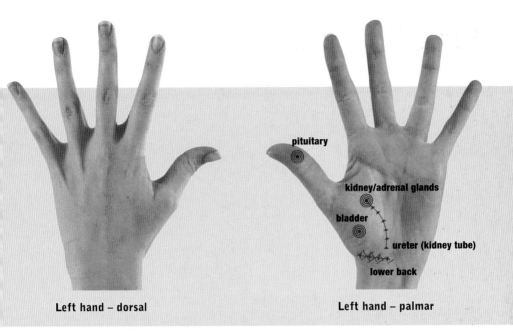

pituitary

kidney/adrenal glands

bladder

ureter (kidney tube)

lower back

Left hand – dorsal

Left hand – palmar

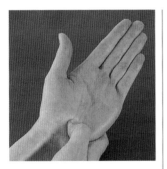

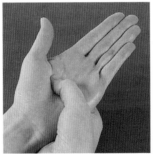

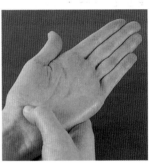

3 Ureter (Kidney tube) reflex

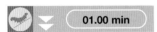 **01.00 min**

Find the base of your lifeline, which starts at the centre of the palm just above the wrist. Use your working thumb to walk along this line and finish when you come to the webbing.

4 Kidney/Adrenal glands reflex

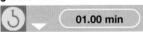 **01.00 min**

Support one hand in the other. Place your working thumb in the webbing between the thumb and index finger just above the thumb muscle halfway down the hand. Use your thumb to hook into the webbing and apply an even pressure.

5 Lower back reflex

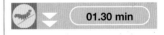 **01.30 min**

Place your working thumb at the base of the hand just above the wrist, and walk along the bone towards the base of the thumb. Make five small steps to the edge of the hand, to represent the five vertebrae in the lumbar spine. Stimulate with small circles at each step.

reproductive conditions

hysterectomy Surgical removal of the womb (uterus) and sometimes ovaries, usually to treat fibroids, cancer of the womb or cervix, heavy menstrual bleeding, endometriosis or prolapse of the womb.

premenstrual syndrome (pms) An imbalance of the sex hormones causing cramps, anxiety, headaches, clumsiness, backache, acne, breast tenderness, depression, insomnia, constipation and/or water retention.

irregular periods Abnormal menstrual bleeding. May result from changes in hormonal activity or may indicate a problem such as fibroids, endometriosis or pelvic inflammatory disease.

pelvic inflammatory disease (pid) Infection of the female internal reproductive organs. The main symptoms are pain and tenderness in the abdomen, fever and backache.

prostatitis Inflammation of the prostate, whose function is to produce lubricating fluid for the sperm during ejaculation. The main symptoms are urine retention and a dull ache between the legs.

To help with these conditions, work on the following reflexes:

Pituitary

Kidney/Adrenal glands

Lower back

Uterus/Prostate

Ovaries/Testicles

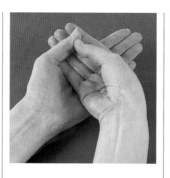

1 Pituitary reflex

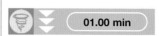 01.00 min

Support one thumb on the fingers of your other hand. Use your working thumb to stimulate the centre of your other thumb.

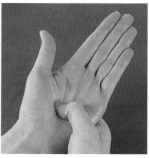

2 Kidney/Adrenal glands reflex

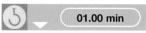 01.00 min

Support one hand in the other. Place your working thumb in the webbing between the thumb and index finger just above the thumb muscle halfway down the hand. Use your thumb to hook into the webbing and apply an even pressure.

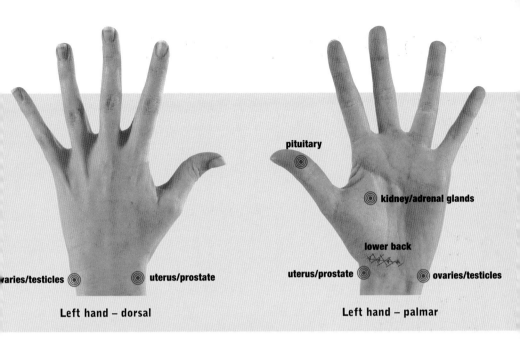

pituitary

kidney/adrenal glands

lower back

ovaries/testicles   uterus/prostate   uterus/prostate   ovaries/testicles

Left hand – dorsal   **Left hand – palmar**

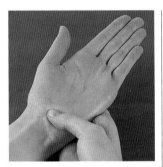

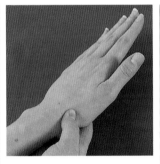

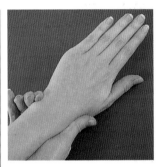

3 Lower back reflex

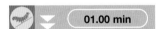 01.00 min

Place your working thumb at the base of the hand just above the wrist, and walk along the bone towards the base of the thumb. Make five small steps to the edge of the hand, to represent the five vertebrae in the lumbar spine. Stimulate with small circles at each step.

4 Uterus/Prostate reflex

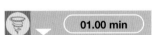 01.00 min

Place your hand palm downward. Use your working thumb to follow down the side of the hand from the thumb and place your tornado at the base of the wrist where you find a small indentation. Apply pressure and stimulate this area.

5 Ovaries/Testicles reflex

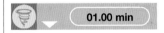 01.00 min

Place your hand palm downward. Use your working index finger to follow down from the little finger and place your tornado at the base of the wrist where you find a small indentation. Apply pressure and stimulate.

treating common conditions 77

balancing the body systems

Treating others: 10-minute treatments

This chapter shows how hand reflexology can be used to create a balanced body system in others. Conditions within each system can be treated so that overall the body can return to a state of wellbeing and harmony.

To treat a partner, ensure that you have created a relaxing environment before you begin. Take your time with each sequence, as all have been designed to be used in an unhurried way – each treatment should take five minutes for each hand.

skin conditions

acne An inflammatory skin condition associated with hormone imbalance during puberty. More common in men, but many women suffer from flare-ups before a period.

boils Round, inflamed, pus-filled lumps on the scalp, face or buttocks or under the arms, resulting from bacterial infection. Symptoms include itching, swelling and pain.

dermatitis Inflammation of the skin that results in itching, thickening, scaling, colour changes and flaking. Often the result of contact with an irritant or allergen.

psoriasis Patches of silvery scales or red areas on the arms, elbows, knees, legs, ears, scalp or back. Toenails and fingernails can sometimes develop ridges.

rosacea Capillaries close to the surface dilate, causing redness and sometimes blotchy red patches, pimples and bumps, generally on the forehead, cheekbones, nose and chin.

To help with these conditions, work on the following reflexes:

Liver/Spleen

Large intestine

Kidney/Adrenal glands

Neck

Pituitary

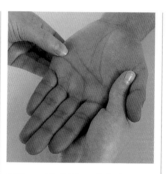

1 Liver (right hand)/Spleen (left hand) reflex

 01.00 min

Place your working thumb on the edge of your partner's hand about one thumbprint down from the base of the little finger. Using the caterpillar walk, take three small steps into the hand. Continue in this manner for five lines, finishing just above the wrist.

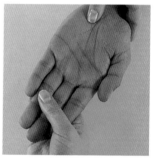

2 Large intestine reflex

 01.30 min

Place your working thumb at the base of zone 4 just above your partner's wrist. Turn your thumbnail so it faces up to the ring finger. Walk up zone 4 until halfway up the hand. Push down and stimulate before turning to walk across the hand, ending up between the webbing.

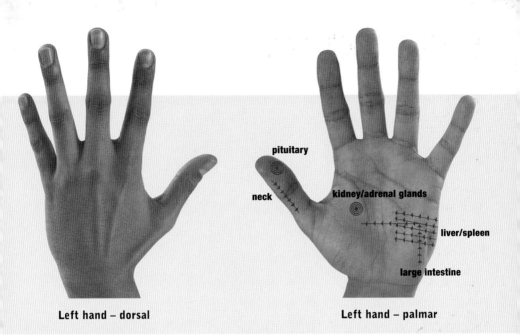

pituitary

neck

kidney/adrenal glands

liver/spleen

large intestine

Left hand – dorsal

Left hand – palmar

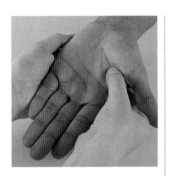

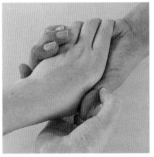

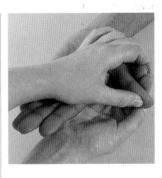

3 Kidney/Adrenal glands reflex

 30 sec

Cradle your partner's hand in your hands. Place your working thumb in the webbing between your partner's thumb and index finger just above the thumb muscle halfway down the hand. Use your thumb to hook into the webbing and apply pressure.

4 Neck reflex

 01.00 min

'Shake hands' with your partner. Use your working thumb to walk along the bone of your partner's thumb from the first to the second joint. Make seven small steps along the bone, to represent the seven vertebrae in the neck. Stimulate with small circles at each step.

5 Pituitary reflex

 01.00 min

Support your partner's hand in the palm of one hand. Use your working thumb to apply pressure and stimulate the centre of your partner's thumb.

muscle strains and tears
Moderate damage to muscle fibres causing bleeding in the muscle tissue. Tenderness and swelling may be accompanied by painful spasms.

muscular dystrophy
A group of rare inherited disorders of unknown cause in which there is a slow but progressive degeneration of the skeletal muscles.

osteoarthritis Characterized by inflammation of a joint, causing creaking, stiffness, swelling, loss of joint function, deformity and pain in most people over the age of 60.

backache Usually caused by muscle strain, although problems in the muscles, ligaments, tendons, bones or in an underlying organ (the kidneys) may also cause it.

slipped disc Extremely painful spinal disorder in which the disc that lies between two vertebrae ruptures so that part of it protrudes.

To help with these conditions, work on the following reflexes:

Parathyroid

Neck

Spine

Knee

Hip

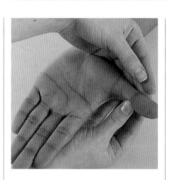

1 Parathyroid reflex

 30 sec

Place your working thumb against the first joint of your partner's thumb. Hook up against the bone on the inside of the thumb just above the webbing and stimulate this area with small clockwise or anticlockwise circles.

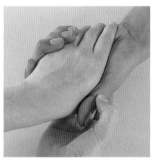

2 Neck reflex

 01.00 min

'Shake hands' with your partner. Use your working thumb to walk along the bone of your partner's thumb from the first to the second joint. Make seven small steps along the bone, to represent the seven vertebrae in the neck. Stimulate with small circles at each step.

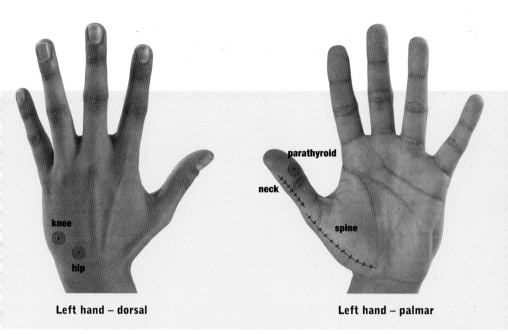

knee

hip

parathyroid

neck

spine

Left hand – dorsal

Left hand – palmar

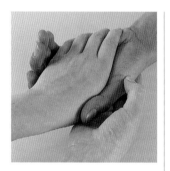

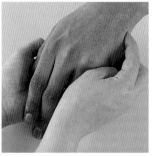

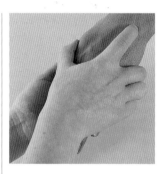

3 Spine reflex

 01.30 min

'Shake hands' with your partner. Use your working thumb to walk along the bone starting at the base of your partner's thumb. Make 12 small steps along the bone to the edge of the wrist. Continue along the bone to the base of the hand.

4 Knee reflex

 01.00 min

Place your partner's hand palm downward and support the hand. Use your working index finger and place it three-quarters of the way down the side of the hand from the little finger. You should find that the bone juts out. Tear against the bone and stimulate.

5 Hip reflex

 01.00 min

Place your partner's hand palm downward and support the hand. Use your working index finger to follow down from the ring finger and, just where the hand meets the wrist, tear back towards the finger and stimulate.

circulatory system

anaemia A lack of red blood cells or haemoglobin. Symptoms include brittle nails, sore mouth or tongue, fatigue and headaches.

angina pectoris Chest pains felt on exertion due to poor blood flow to the heart muscle.

atherosclerosis Fat deposits build up on the lining of the walls of the arteries, making them harder and narrower, and impede blood flow. Symptoms can include chest pain and shortness of breath.

high blood pressure (hypertension) This rarely causes any symptoms. Warning signs associated with advanced hypertension include headaches, shortness of breath, visual disturbances and dizziness.

deep vein thrombosis (dvt) A serious condition affecting the deep-lying veins in the legs. Symptoms include swelling, reddish skin discolouration and pain.

To help with these conditions, work on the following reflexes:

Diaphragm

Heart

Cardiac

Kidney/Adrenal glands

Liver/Spleen

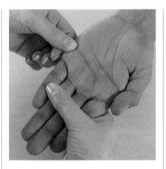

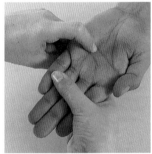

1 Diaphragm reflex

  01.00 min

Place your working thumb a third of the way down your partner's palm. Use the butterfly movement to walk across the hand from one side to the other.

2 Heart reflex

  01.00 min

Place your working thumb on the diaphragm line in zone 4 of your partner's palm. Take a half thumbprint step towards the wrist. Hook up towards the little finger and stimulate with small circles.

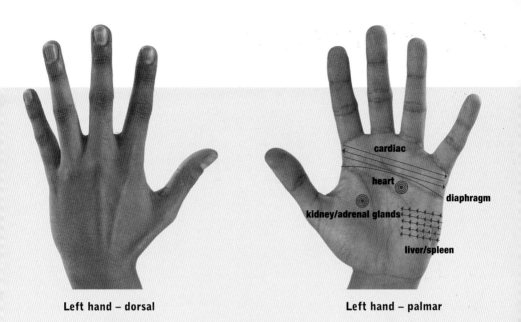

Left hand – dorsal

Left hand – palmar

cardiac
heart
diaphragm
kidney/adrenal glands
liver/spleen

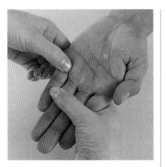

3 Cardiac reflex

 01.00 min

Use your working thumb to walk across your partner's hand from the base of the fingers to the diaphragm line.

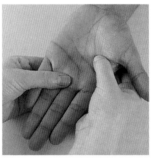

4 Kidney/Adrenal glands reflex

 01.00 min

Cradle your partner's hand in your hands. Place your working thumb in the webbing between your partner's thumb and index finger just above the thumb muscle halfway down the hand. Use your thumb to hook into the webbing and apply pressure.

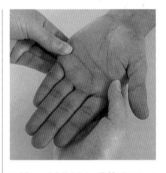

5 Liver (right hand)/Spleen (left hand) reflex

 01.00 min

Place your working thumb on the edge of your partner's hand about one thumbprint down from the base of the little finger. Using the caterpillar walk, take three small steps into the hand. Continue in this manner for five lines, finishing just above the wrist.

immune system

myalgic encephalomyelitis (me) Serious viral infection or damage to the immune system is a possible cause. Symptoms include severe debilitating muscle fatigue, headaches, dizziness, depression and panic states.

bacterial infections Most bacteria are harmless to humans, but produce poisons that can be harmful in large quantities. Antibiotics usually cure bacterial infections.

fungal infections Characterized by moist, possibly itchy, red patches anywhere on the body, these can be produced in the skin and/or mucous membranes.

allergies The result of inappropriate responses by the body's immune system to a substance that is not normally harmful (an allergen).

rheumatoid arthritis The body is attacked by its own immune system, causing inflammation and damage or destruction of the cartilage and tissues around the joints. Symptoms include aching or stiffness of the joints, which is worse in the morning and lasts for several hours.

To help with these conditions, work on the following reflexes:

Liver/Spleen

Lungs

Kidney/Adrenal glands

Large intestine

Lymphatics

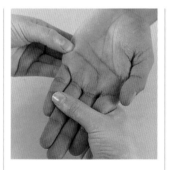

1 Liver (right hand)/Spleen (left hand) reflex

 01.00 min

Place your working thumb on the edge of your partner's hand about one thumbprint down from the base of the little finger. Using the caterpillar walk, take three small steps into the hand. Continue in this manner for five lines, finishing just above the wrist.

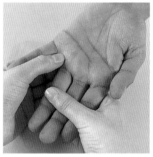

2 Lungs reflex

 01.00 min

Place your working thumb halfway down the palm of your partner's hand between zones 5 and 4. Apply pressure and caterpillar walk towards the base of the fingers and between the bones. Continue in this manner between zones 4 and 3 and zones 3 and 2.

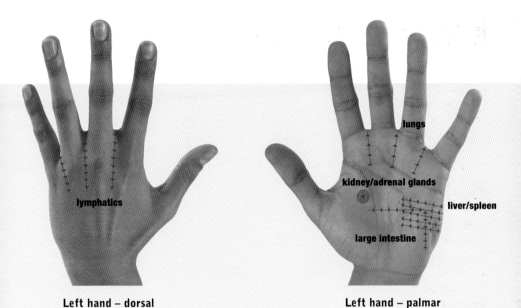

lungs

kidney/adrenal glands

lymphatics

liver/spleen

large intestine

Left hand – dorsal

Left hand – palmar

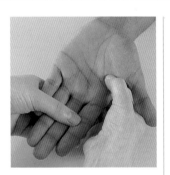

3 Kidney/Adrenal glands reflex

 01.00 min

Cradle your partner's hand in your hands. Place your working thumb in the webbing between your partner's thumb and index finger just above the thumb muscle halfway down the hand. Use your thumb to hook into the webbing and apply pressure.

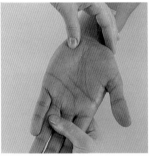

4 Large intestine reflex

 01.00 min

Place your working thumb at the base of zone 4 just above your partner's wrist. Turn your thumbnail so it faces up to the ring finger. Walk up zone 4 until halfway up the hand. Push down and stimulate before turning to walk across the hand, ending up between the webbing.

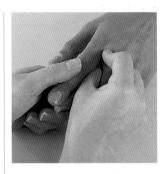

5 Lymphatics reflex

 01.00 min

Place your partner's hand palm downward. Place your working index finger and thumb between the bases of the index and middle fingers. Apply pressure and, using bird's beak, take tiny steps towards the wrist. Continue in this manner between zones 3 and 4 and zones 4 and 5.

nervous system

facial palsy Condition, often temporary and with no known cause, characterized by the eyelid and the corner of the mouth drooping on one side.

meniere's disease Inner ear disorder caused by build-up of fluid in the canals controlling balance. The main symptoms are frequent severe, sudden vertigo, tinnitus and deafness.

multiple sclerosis Debilitating disease that damages the nerve fibres in the brain and spinal cord. Symptoms include blurred vision, slurred speech and muscle weakness.

parkinson's disease The result of damage to nerve cells in the base of the brain. Symptoms are muscle tremors, weakness and stiffness.

paralysis The partial or complete, temporary or permanent, loss of controlled movement in any muscles of the body. May also include loss of feeling.

To help with these conditions, work on the following reflexes:

Hypothalamus

Inner ear/Balance

Neck

Spine

Sciatic

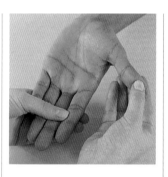

1 Hypothalamus reflex

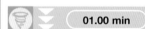 01.00 min

Support your partner's hand in the palm of your hand. Use your working thumb to stimulate the outside edge of your partner's thumb.

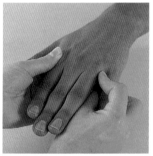

2 Inner ear/Balance reflex

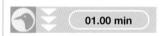 01.00 min

Place your partner's hand palm downward and support it. Place your working index finger and thumb on the joint at the base of the ring finger. Apply pressure and make small circles to stimulate this area.

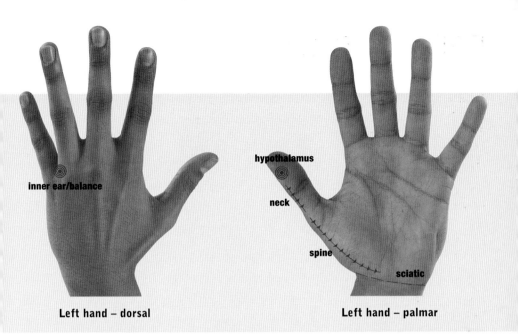

inner ear/balance

hypothalamus

neck

spine

sciatic

Left hand – dorsal

Left hand – palmar

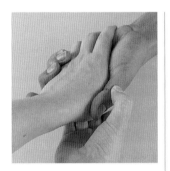

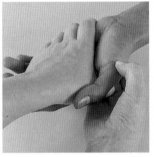

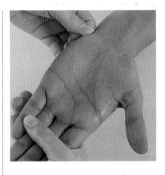

3 Neck reflex

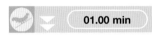 01.00 min

4 Spine reflex

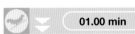 01.00 min

5 Sciatic reflex

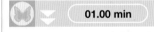 01.00 min

'Shake hands' with your partner. Use your working thumb to walk along the bone of your partner's thumb from the first to the second joint. Make seven small steps along the bone, to represent the seven vertebrae in the neck. Stimulate with small circles at each step.

'Shake hands' with your partner. Use your working thumb to walk along the bone, starting at the base of your partner's thumb. Make 12 small steps along the bone to the edge of the wrist. Continue along the bone to the base of the hand.

Place your working thumb at the base of your partner's hand where it meets the wrist. Walk across the top of the wrist using the butterfly technique.

endocrine system

diabetes mellitus A reduction in insulin production by the pancreas results in high blood-sugar levels. Symptoms include frequent urination, irritability, abnormal thirst and weakness.

adrenal insufficiency
Underproduction of the hormone cortisol by the adrenal glands. Symptoms may include weakness, fatigue, abdominal pain, nausea, dehydration and deepening of skin colour.

underactive thyroid (hypothyroidism)
Underproduction of the hormone thyroxine, which helps regulate energy levels. Symptoms may include loss of appetite, weight increase, inability to tolerate cold, and fatigue.

overactive thyroid (hyperthyroidism) Levels of thyroid hormones in the blood are excessively high. Symptoms may include weight loss, nervousness, excessive sweating and a swelling in the neck.

enlarged prostate The gradual enlargement (non-cancerous) of the prostate largely due to hormonal changes. Urination becomes difficult and painful. May cause bladder infections.

To help with these conditions, work on the following reflexes:

Pituitary

Thyroid

Pancreas

Kidney/Adrenal glands

Uterus/Prostate and Ovaries/Testicles

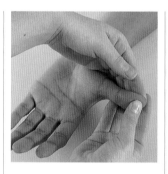

1 Pituitary reflex

 01.00 min

Place your partner's hand palm upward. Use your working thumb to apply pressure and to stimulate the centre of your partner's thumb.

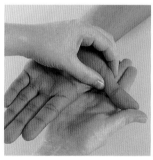

2 Thyroid reflex

 01.00 min

Support your partner's thumb on the fingers of one hand. Use your working thumb to walk up from the base of the thumb to the first crease; you should be stimulating the half of the thumb that is closest to the index finger.

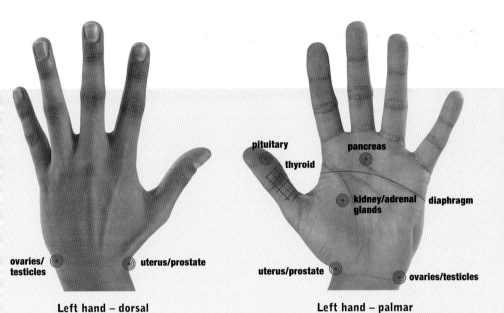

pituitary
thyroid
pancreas
kidney/adrenal glands
diaphragm
ovaries/testicles
uterus/prostate
uterus/prostate
ovaries/testicles

Left hand – dorsal

Left hand – palmar

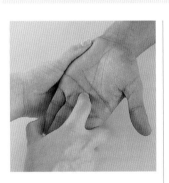

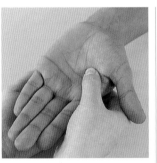

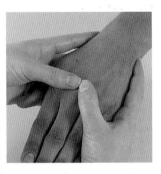

3 Pancreas reflex

  01.00 min

Place your working index finger on the diaphragm line at the joint at the base of your partner's middle finger. Hook up towards the middle finger and against the joint and stimulate by making small circles.

4 Kidney/Adrenal glands reflex

01.00 min

Cradle your partner's hand in your hands. Place your working thumb in the webbing between your partner's thumb and index finger just above the thumb muscle halfway down the hand. Use your thumb to hook into the webbing and apply pressure.

5 Uterus/Prostate and Ovaries/Testicles

 01.00 min

Place your partner's hand palm downward. Using both your index fingers, follow down from your partner's little finger and thumb so that they are on either side of the wrist. Apply pressure at the base of the wrist where you find the small indentations and stimulate this area.

respiratory system

asthma Recurrent episodes of breathlessness caused by constricted airways. An increase of mucus and inflammation in the lungs makes it hard to breathe.

emphysema Disease in which the tiny air sacs (alveoli) of the lungs become damaged, causing a progressively worsening and incurable shortness of breath.

bronchitis The tubes (bronchi) that lead to the lungs become inflamed or obstructed, leading to excess mucus, fever, coughing, sore throat and breathing difficulty.

upper respiratory infections Infection, caused by viruses or bacteria, results in inflammation and swelling of the mucous membranes lining the sinuses and/or throat.

sinusitis Inflammation of the facial sinuses caused by an allergy or infection with bacteria or viruses. Pressure inside the sinuses causes pain and fever.

To help with these conditions, work on the following reflexes:

Sinuses

Diaphragm

Lungs

Nose

Lymphatics

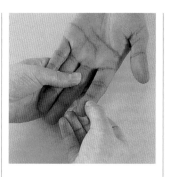

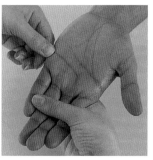

1 Sinuses reflex

 | 01.00 min

Support your partner's fingers in one hand. Use your working thumb to walk from the tip to the base, or the base to the tip, of one finger. Continue in this manner until you have worked all the fingers. Stimulate with tiny circles at each step.

2 Diaphragm reflex

 | 01.00 min

Place your working thumb a third of the way down your partner's palm. Use the butterfly movement to walk across the hand from one side to the other.

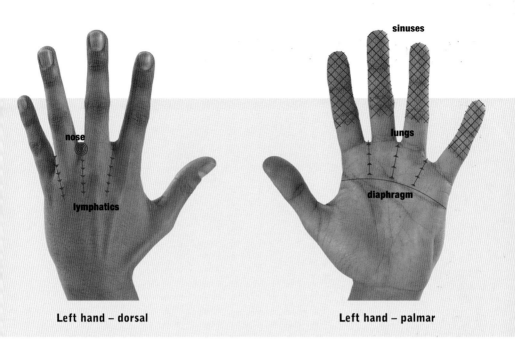

sinuses

nose

lungs

lymphatics

diaphragm

Left hand – dorsal

Left hand – palmar

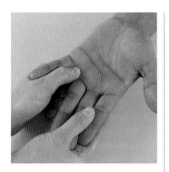

3 Lungs reflex

 01.00 min

Place your working thumb halfway down the palm of your partner's hand between zones 5 and 4. Apply pressure and caterpillar walk towards the base of the fingers and between the bones. Continue in this manner between zones 4 and 3 and zones 3 and 2.

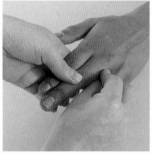

4 Nose reflex

 01.00 min

Place your partner's hand palm downward. Use your working index finger and thumb to stimulate deep in the webbing between your partner's middle and ring fingers.

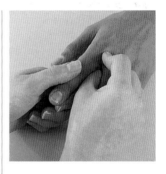

5 Lymphatics reflex

 01.00 min

Place your partner's hand palm downward. Place your working index finger and thumb between the bases of the index and middle fingers. Apply pressure and, using bird's beak, take tiny steps towards the wrist. Continue in this manner between zones 3 and 4 and zones 4 and 5.

digestive system

constipation Infrequent, painful or difficult passing of hard, dry faeces, usually due to insufficient fibre and fluid in the diet.

crohn's disease Ulceration of a section or sections of the digestive tract anywhere from mouth to anus. The passageway narrows as it heals, causing pain. Symptoms include severe abdominal pain and rectal bleeding.

diverticulitis Inflammation of colon lining resulting in pouch-like areas (diverticula) forming. They can trap waste matter, causing cramping, bloating, constipation or diarrhoea, and nausea.

gall bladder disorders Usually the result of gall stones, causing extreme pain in the upper right abdomen, accompanied by vomiting, fever and nausea.

haemorrhoids Swollen veins in the rectum, which may protrude from the anus. Common symptoms include bleeding, itching, pain, burning and swelling.

To help with these conditions, work on the following reflexes:

Gall bladder

Liver/Spleen

Kidney/Adrenal glands

Large intestine

Pancreas

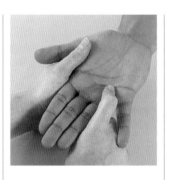

1 Gall bladder reflex

 01.00 min

Place your working thumb on the diaphragm line at the joint at the base of your partner's ring finger. Hook up towards the ring finger and stimulate with tiny circles against the joint.

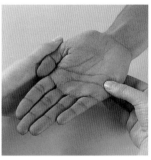

2 Liver (right hand)/Spleen (left hand) reflex

 01.00 min

Place your working thumb on the edge of your partner's hand about one thumbprint down from the base of the little finger. Using the caterpillar walk, take three small steps into the hand. Continue in this manner for five lines, finishing just above the wrist.

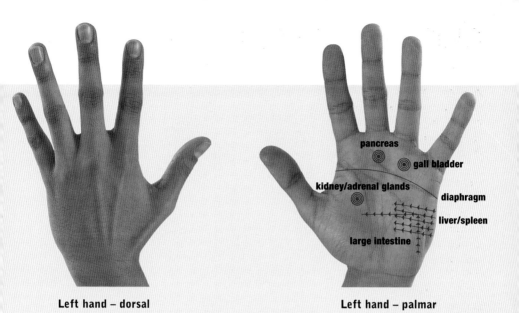

Left hand – dorsal

Left hand – palmar

pancreas
gall bladder
kidney/adrenal glands
diaphragm
liver/spleen
large intestine

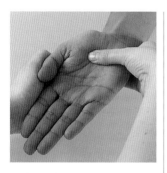

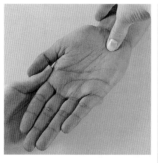

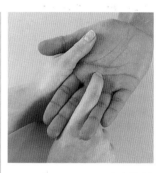

3 Kidney/Adrenal glands reflex

 01.00 min

Cradle your partner's hand in your hands. Place your working thumb in the webbing between your partner's thumb and index finger just above the thumb muscle halfway down the hand. Use your thumb to hook into the webbing and apply pressure.

4 Large intestine reflex

 01.00 min

Place your working thumb at the base of zone 4 just above your partner's wrist. Turn your thumbnail so it faces up to the ring finger. Walk up zone 4 until halfway up the hand. Push down and stimulate before turning to walk across the hand, ending up between the webbing.

5 Pancreas reflex

 01.00 min

Place your working index finger on the diaphragm line at the joint at the base of your partner's middle finger. Hook up towards the middle finger and against the joint and stimulate by making small circles.

urinary system

polycystic kidneys A rare inherited disorder in which numerous cysts develop in both kidneys, gradually increasing in size and destroying most normal kidney tissue.

kidney infection Often occurs as a result of bacteria ascending to the kidneys from the bladder. Symptoms may include backache, chills and fever.

cystitis Bacterial infection of the bladder resulting in inflammation. Symptoms can include painful urination, frequent and urgent desire to urinate, and possibly blood in the urine.

bed-wetting Involuntary urinating in bed, common in early childhood and also occurs in the elderly.

incontinence The inability to control urination (passage of urine). Urinary incontinence can range from an occasional leakage of urine to a complete inability to hold any urine.

To help with these conditions, work on the following reflexes:

Pituitary/Hypothalamus

Bladder

Ureter (Kidney tube)

Kidney/Adrenal glands

Lower back

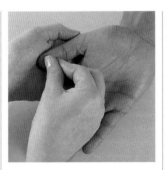

1 Pituitary/Hypothalamus reflexes

 01.00 min

Support your partner's hand in the palm of your hand. Use your working thumb and index finger to simultaneously stimulate the centre and the outside edge of your partner's thumb.

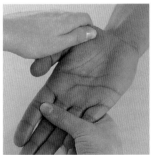

2 Bladder reflex

 30 sec

Place your working thumb in the base of the muscle of your partner's thumb. Tear down towards the wrist and stimulate.

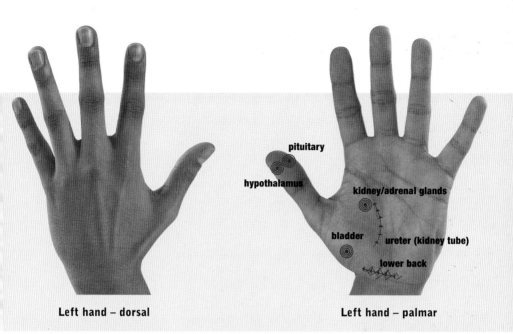

pituitary

hypothalamus

kidney/adrenal glands

bladder

ureter (kidney tube)

lower back

Left hand – dorsal

Left hand – palmar

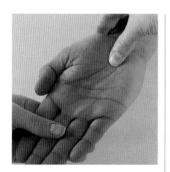

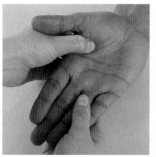

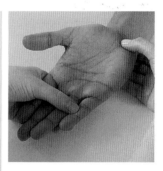

3 Ureter (Kidney tube) reflex

01.00 min

Support your partner's hand. Place your working thumb at the base of the wrist where the lifeline begins. Apply pressure to this area and walk up the lifeline, finishing when you come to the webbing.

4 Kidney/Adrenal glands reflex

01.00 min

Cradle your partner's hand in your hands. Place your working thumb in the webbing between your partner's thumb and index finger just above the thumb muscle halfway down the hand. Use your thumb to hook into the webbing and apply pressure.

5 Lower back reflex

01.30 min

Place your working thumb at the base of your partner's hand just above the wrist, and walk along the bone towards the base of the thumb. Make five small steps to the edge of the hand, to represent the five vertebrae in the lumbar spine. Stimulate with small circles at each step.

reproductive system

impotence in men
Characterized by an inability to achieve or sustain an erection adequate for sexual intercourse.

infertility in men
Pin-pointing the exact problem is difficult, although most often it is the result of low numbers of sperm or abnormal sperm.

infertility in women
Failure to conceive after a year or more of regular sexual activity during ovulation.

prolapse of the womb
Develops when the pelvic muscles become injured or weakened so that they can no longer hold the womb in place. Symptoms can include backache, abdominal discomfort, heavy periods and urinary incontinence.

endometriosis
A condition in which cells from the womb lining find their way out of the womb and grow in different areas of the body. Symptoms can include heavy bleeding, painful periods and lower back pain.

To help with these conditions, work on the following reflexes:

Uterus/Prostate and Ovaries/Testicles

Penis

Pituitary

Lower back

Fallopian tube/Vas deferens

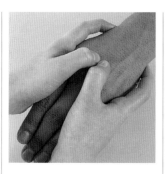

1 Uterus/Prostate and Ovaries/Testicles reflexes

 01.00 min

Place your partner's hand palm downward. Use both your index fingers to follow down from your partner's little finger and thumb so that your fingers are on either side of the wrist. Apply pressure at the base of the wrist where you find the small indentations and stimulate this area.

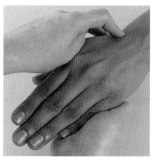

2 Penis reflex

 30 sec

From the prostate reflex point use your working index finger to take one small step towards the top of your partner's hand. Push in and tear down towards the prostate reflex.

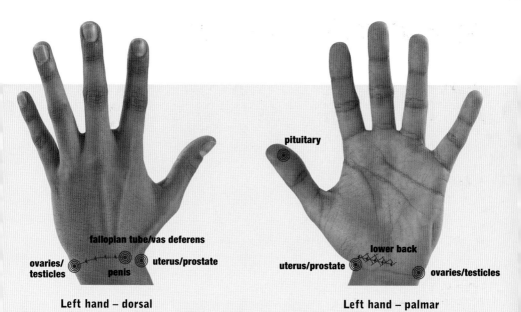

pituitary

fallopian tube/vas deferens

ovaries/testicles

penis

uterus/prostate

Left hand – dorsal

lower back

uterus/prostate

ovaries/testicles

Left hand – palmar

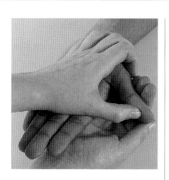

3 Pituitary reflex

01.00 min

Support your partner's hand in the palm of your hand. Use your working thumb to apply pressure and stimulate the centre of your partner's thumb.

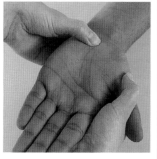

4 Lower back reflex

01.30 min

Place your working thumb at the base of your partner's hand just above the wrist, and walk along the bone towards the base of the thumb. Make five small steps to the edge of the hand, to represent the five vertebrae in the lumbar spine. Stimulate with small circles at each step.

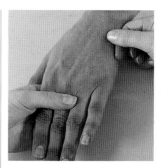

5 Fallopian tube/ Vas deferens reflex

01.00 min

Place your partner's hand palm downward. Use your working thumb to walk across the area where the wrist meets the hand, joining the ovaries/testicles and uterus/prostate reflexes.

specialized hand reflexology

Treating yourself and others: 15-minute treatments

This chapter shows how hand reflexology can be used to help with particular stages in our lives, from pregnancy to menopause, or to combat stress. Each sequence can be used to treat yourself or others and should take a total of 15 minutes – follow the 'Using this seqence' text to maximize the benefits of each session.

pregnancy, weeks 14–36

dizziness Common after about 16 weeks, and caused by a drop in blood pressure as the expanding womb starts to push against the major blood vessels.

constipation Common during pregnancy when food moves more slowly through the intestines because of hormonal changes affecting certain muscles. Iron supplements make it worse.

carpal tunnel syndrome Compression of nerves in the wrist (see also page 66), characterized by numb, tingling and painful fingers. Fairly common in late stages of pregnancy.

oedema The retention of water or body fluid, which causes the soft tissues to swell. The fingers, legs, ankles and feet become slightly puffy and uncomfortable.

Using this sequence

Most pregnancy-associated problems are the result of hormonal changes, vitamin and mineral deficiencies, and a redistribution of weight because of weight gain. After week 14, reflexology can help to relieve these problems, and restore homoeostasis (natural balance). Practise the sequence once a day.

To help with these conditions, work on the following reflexes:

Eustachian tube

Stomach

Large intestine

Carpal tunnel

Urethra

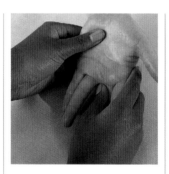

1 Eustachian tube reflex

 ⌄⌄⌄ (01.00 min)

Support your partner's hand. Place your working thumb between the middle and ring fingers. Apply pressure and tear towards the joint at the base of the middle finger and stimulate with small circles.

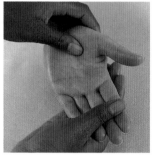

2 Stomach reflex

 ⌄⌄⌄ (01.30 min)

Support your partner's hand. Place your working thumb at the tip of the webbing between the thumb and index finger, then walk to the edge of the hand and return back to your original point. Continue until you have covered the webbing, rather like the spokes of a bicycle wheel.

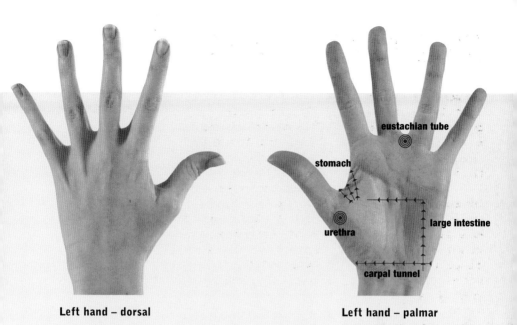

eustachian tube

stomach

urethra

large intestine

carpal tunnel

Left hand – dorsal   **Left hand – palmar**

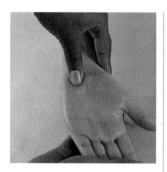

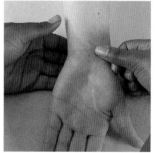

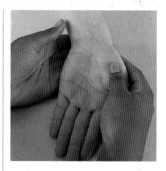

3 Large intestine reflex

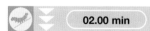 02.00 min

Place your working thumb at the base of zone 4 just above your partner's wrist. Turn your thumbnail so it faces up to the ring finger. Walk up zone 4 until halfway up the hand. Push down and stimulate before turning to walk across the hand, ending up between the webbing.

4 Carpal tunnel reflex

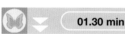 01.30 min

Support your partner's hand palm upward. Place your working thumb at one side of the wrist and butterfly walk across the hand from one side of the wrist to the other. Stimulate with small circles at each step. Repeat.

5 Urethra reflex

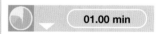 01.00 min

Place your working thumb at the base of your partner's thumb. Tear down into the muscle and towards the wrist and stimulate.

pregnancy, weeks 37–40

mood changes Common during pregnancy, these are often caused by hormonal changes and vitamin B deficiencies, and physical and psychological stress.

backache The root of this common problem is often poor posture; also weight gain and the muscle-relaxing effects of the hormone progesterone.

insomnia Very common during the final weeks of pregnancy, it is linked to low vitamin B levels, difficulty in getting comfortable and anxiety about the birth.

induced labour Synthetic oxytocin is used to induce labour and sometimes to expel the placenta after delivery.

post-natal depression Characterized by overwhelming and debilitating listlessness, making the simple tasks associated with life in general or the baby hard to cope with.

Using this sequence
Work towards a natural birth by practising this sequence daily, and as you get closer to term, twice daily, applying more pressure to the pituitary reflex. This gland produces oxytocin, the hormone that makes the womb contract in labour and stimulates breast milk. Continue the sequence daily after birth, to work towards rebalancing your hormones and overcoming post-natal depression.

To help with these conditions, work on the following reflexes:

Pituitary/Oxytocin

Thyroid

Uterus and Ovaries

Spine

Kidney/Adrenal glands

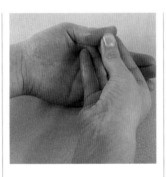

1 Pituitary/Oxytocin reflex

 02.00 min

Support one thumb on the fingers of your other hand. Use your working thumb to apply pressure and stimulate the centre of the thumb.

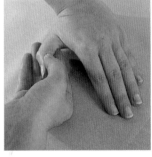

2 Thyroid reflex

 01.00 min

Place your hand palm downward and support one thumb in the other hand. Use your working thumb to walk between the two creases of the thumb. You should be stimulating the half of the thumb that is closest to the index finger.

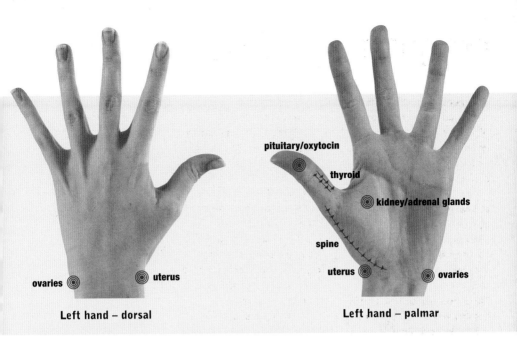

pituitary/oxytocin
thyroid
kidney/adrenal glands
spine
uterus
ovaries

ovaries
uterus

Left hand – dorsal

Left hand – palmar

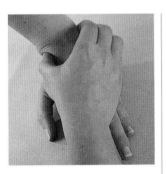

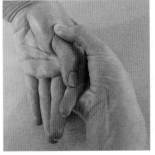

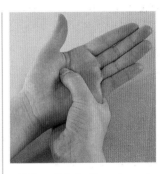

3 Uterus and Ovaries reflex

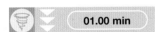 01.00 min

Turn your hand palm downward. Use your working thumb and index finger to follow down from your thumb and little finger. At either side of the base of the wrist you will find a small indentation. Apply pressure and stimulate.

4 Spine reflex

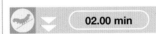 02.00 min

Cradle one hand in the other. Use your working thumb to walk along the bone, starting at the base of the thumb. Make 12 small steps along the bone to the edge of the wrist. Continue along the bone to the base of the hand.

5 Kidney/Adrenal glands reflex

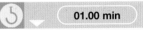 01.00 min

Support one hand in the other. Place your working thumb in the webbing between the thumb and index finger just above the thumb muscle halfway down the hand. Use your thumb to hook into the webbing and apply pressure.

babies

Babies enjoy gentle hand reflexology as they are highly receptive to touch and therapeutic stimuli. Each technique has different beneficial effects on a baby and any underlying tensions need to be sensitively explored as his/her needs will change each day.

Your touch can help your baby experience pleasure, enhance non-verbal communication and give him/her a sense of safety, wellbeing and balance. Reflexology can help your baby to release tension after the birth and to adjust to life in the outside world. Over time, reflexology can assist in building up a healthy immune system and balancing the energies in all the body's systems, aiding proper functioning.

Using this sequence

Practise this treatment daily when your baby has been fed. Put him/her on a bed or the floor in a warm room with low lighting and relaxing music. Use cornstarch or sweet almond oil to reduce friction. Begin with a light touch and increase the pressure as your baby gets used to the reflexology and your confidence increases. Keep sessions brief for newborns as they have a short attention span.

To help with these conditions, work on the following reflexes:

Sinuses

Eustachian tube

Liver/Spleen

Intestines

Lymphatics

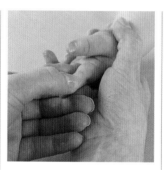

1 Sinuses reflex

 02.00 min

Support your baby's fingers in one hand. Use your working thumb to walk from the base to the tip, or the tip to the base, of a finger. Continue in this manner until you have worked all the fingers. Stimulate with tiny circles at each step.

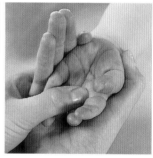

2 Eustachian tube reflex

 01.00 min

Support your baby's hand in yours. Place your working thumb between the middle and ring fingers and stimulate the area with small circles.

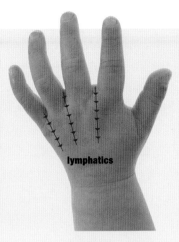

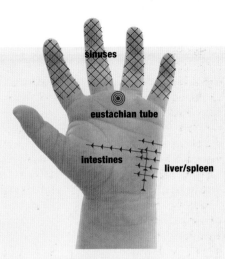

sinuses

eustachian tube

intestines

liver/spleen

lymphatics

Left hand – dorsal

Left hand – palmar

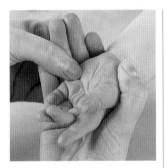

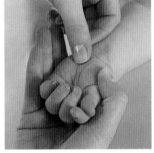

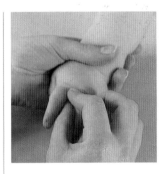

3 Liver (right hand)/Spleen (left hand) reflex

 01.00 min

Place your working thumb on the edge of your baby's hand about one thumbprint down from the base of the little finger. Using the caterpillar walk, take three small steps into the hand. Continue in this manner for five lines, finishing just above the wrist.

4 Intestines reflex

 02.00 min

Place your working thumb at the base of zone 4 just above your baby's wrist. Turn your thumbnail so it faces up to the ring finger. Walk up zone 4 until halfway up the hand. Stimulate before turning to walk across the hand, ending up between the webbing.

5 Lymphatics reflex

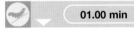 01.00 min

Place your baby's hand palm downward. Place your working index finger and thumb between the bases of the index and middle fingers. Using bird's beak, take tiny steps towards the wrist. Continue in this manner between zones 3 and 4 and zones 4 and 5.

specialized hand reflexology 107

young children

Hand reflexology can help to stimulate the healing processes as well as ensuring that all body systems are functioning on every level. Remember – any child who develops a medical problem should be taken to a doctor or to a hospital emergency department as soon as possible.

poor appetite Usually a sign or symptom of some other problem. May be caused by emotional factors (stress, anxiety, depression) or a nutritional deficiency.

croup Respiratory infection that causes narrowing of the throat due to swelling. Mucus may increase and clog up the airways. Symptoms include difficulty breathing and a barking cough.

hyperactivity Medically termed attention deficit and hyperactivity disorder (ADHD). Mainly affecting children, it is characterized by behavioural problems.

Using this sequence

Perform this treatment in a quiet room, with low lighting, no telephones and tranquil music, preferably in the evening just before or after a bedtime story. Make sure your child is comfortable and can fall asleep if necessary. Put any toys or comforters within easy reach.

To help with these conditions, work on the following reflexes:

Lungs

Throat

Intestines

Kidney/Adrenal glands

Spine

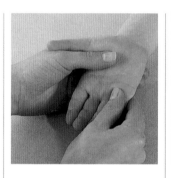

1 Lungs reflex

 01.00 min

Place your working thumb halfway down the palm of your child's hand between zones 5 and 4. Apply pressure and use the caterpillar walk towards the base of the fingers and between the bones. Continue in this manner between zones 4 and 3 and zones 3 and 2.

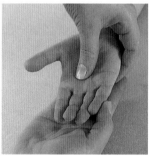

2 Throat reflex

 01.00 min

Place your working thumb one third of the way down your child's hand between the index and middle fingers. Slowly walk up between the bones to the bases of the first and second fingers. Repeat, stimulating with small circles at each step.

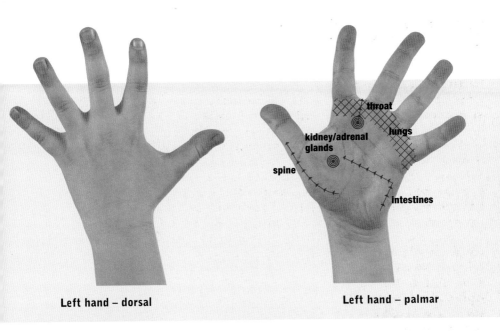

Left hand – dorsal

Left hand – palmar

throat
kidney/adrenal glands
lungs
spine
intestines

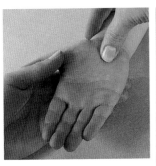

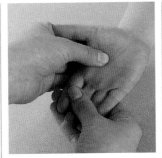

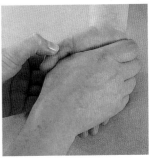

3 Intestines reflex

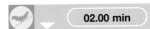 02.00 min

Place your working thumb at the base of zone 4 just above your child's wrist. Turn your thumbnail so it faces up to the ring finger. Walk up zone 4 until halfway up the hand. Stimulate before turning to walk across the hand, ending up between the webbing.

4 Kidney/Adrenal glands reflex

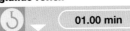 01.00 min

Cradle your child's hand in your hands. Place your working thumb in the webbing between the child's thumb and index finger just above the thumb muscle halfway down the hand. Use your thumb to hook into the webbing and apply light pressure.

5 Spine reflex

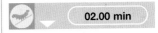 02.00 min

'Shake hands' with your child. Use your working thumb to walk along the bone of the thumb from the first to the second joint, then from the second joint to the base of the hand.

menopause

Menopause occurs once a woman stops producing eggs and her periods cease, indicating the end of fertility, usually between the ages of 51 and 55. The ovaries also produce smaller amounts of the sex hormones, oestrogen and progesterone, causing the physiological and many of the psychological changes.

Symptoms experienced include mood swings, depression, headaches, dizziness, fatigue, night sweats, bladder problems, breast tenderness, ageing skin, insomnia, vaginal dryness, discomfort during sexual intercourse, lack of interest in sex and, of course, hot flushes.

After the menopause there may be increased risk of osteoporosis, heart disease and hypothyroidism or underactive thyroid (see also page 90).

Using this sequence
Daily use of the treatment below will help to minimize many of the unpleasant side-effects that are associated with the menopause.

To help with these conditions, work on the following reflexes:

Spine

Pituitary

Parathyroid

Kidney/Adrenal glands

Ovaries

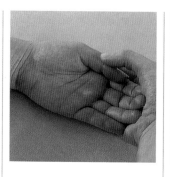

1 Spine reflex

 03.00 min

Cup one hand in the other so that your thumb is resting between your index and middle fingers. Use your working thumb to walk along the bone of the supported thumb from the first to the second joint. Continue to walk along the bone from the second joint to the base of the hand.

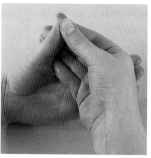

2 Pituitary reflex

 01.00 min

Support one thumb on the fingers of your other hand. Use your working thumb to apply pressure and stimulate the centre of your other thumb.

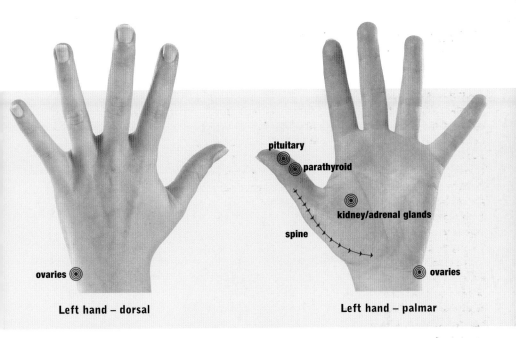

pituitary
parathyroid
kidney/adrenal glands
spine
ovaries
ovaries

Left hand – dorsal

Left hand – palmar

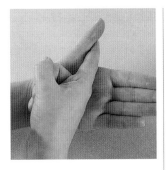

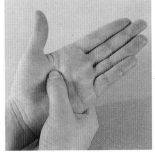

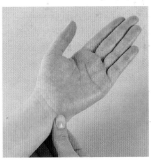

3 Parathyroid reflex

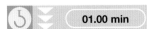

01.00 min

Support your thumb as shown. Place your working index finger against the first joint of the inner section of the thumb. Hook up against the bone and stimulate this area in clockwise or anticlockwise circles.

4 Kidney/Adrenal glands reflex

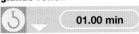

01.00 min

Support one hand in the other. Place your working thumb in the webbing between the thumb and index finger just above the thumb muscle halfway down the hand. Use your thumb to hook into the webbing and apply an even pressure.

5 Ovaries reflex

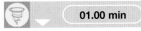

01.00 min

Place your hand palm upward. Use your working index finger to follow down from the little finger and place your tornado at the base of the wrist where you find a small indentation. Apply pressure and stimulate.

golden years

As people grow older, their immune systems deteriorate, making them more susceptible to disease. Ageing is a natural process, and so is slowing down, because the body is becoming weaker.

One of the most common conditions found in the elderly is arthritis or joint disease. Inflammation of one or more joints is characterized by stiffness, pain and swelling. There is often a diminished range of movements and, in most cases, a usual pattern of morning pain and stiffness.

Hand reflexology is a very effective treatment for the elderly, helping with many aches and pains and relieving the symptoms of chronic ailments. On the most basic level, reflexology can increase the circulation, which is important for older people.

Using this sequence

Practise this treatment daily, or even twice daily if necessary. Be careful to work lightly over areas of loose skin and broken blood vessels, and to work with the natural configuration of the fingers. Older joints can be brittle and less flexible than younger ones. The overall pressure should be light and should not cause discomfort; if it does, then reduce the pressure to a comfortable level.

To help with these conditions, work on the following reflexes:

Head

Bladder

Liver/Spleen

Large intestine

Lymphatics

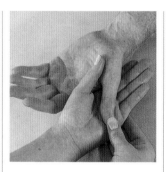

1 Head reflex

 02.00 min

Cradle your partner's thumb in your fingers. Use your working thumb to walk from the tip to the base of the thumb. Continue in this manner until you have covered the entire thumb. Stimulate with tiny circles at each step.

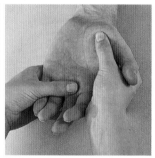

2 Bladder reflex

 01.00 min

Place your working thumb in the base of the muscle of your partner's thumb. Tear down towards the wrist and stimulate.

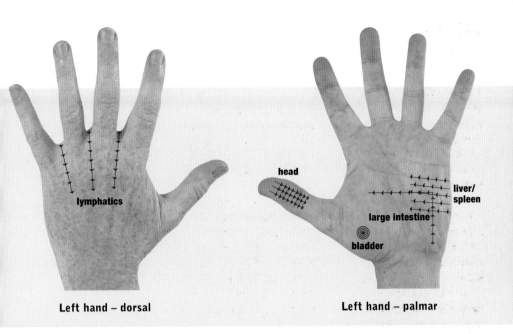

lymphatics

head

liver/spleen

large intestine

bladder

Left hand – dorsal

Left hand – palmar

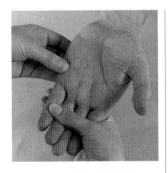

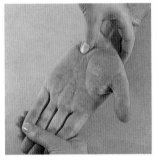

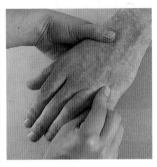

3 Liver (right hand)/Spleen (left hand) reflex

 01.00 min

Place your working thumb on the edge of your partner's hand about one thumbprint down from the base of the little finger. Using the caterpillar walk, take three small steps into the hand. Continue in this manner for five lines, finishing just above the wrist.

4 Large intestine reflex

 02.00 min

Place your working thumb at the base of zone 4 just above your partner's wrist. Turn your thumbnail so it faces up to the ring finger. Walk up zone 4 until halfway up the hand. Push down and stimulate before turning to walk across the hand, ending up between the webbing.

5 Lymphatics reflex

 01.00 min

Place your partner's hand palm downward. Place your working index finger and thumb between the bases of the ring and little fingers. Using bird's beak, take tiny steps towards the wrist. Continue in this manner between zones 3 and 4 and zones 2 and 3.

terminal illness

Hand reflexology can treat the stress around many terminal illnesses, helping to control the pain and improve the patient's general condition and quality of life on a day-to-day basis. Treatment encourages the production of endorphins, which can inhibit the transmission of pain and help the body to relax. Medication often causes a range of unpleasant side-effects and hand reflexology can help the body deal with these and achieve balance.

Reflexology can also offer a sensitive, non-verbal means of expressing love. It can give a reason for visiting, it can take the mind off pain and suffering and it is something positive to do.

Using this sequence

Apply the treatment as many times as you feel necessary throughout the day. It is important to use gentle pressure, adjusting it in order to avoid discomfort and make sure each treatment is pleasurable. The treatment can be given while the person is sitting up or while lying in bed, in which case they can fall asleep whenever they wish.

To help with these conditions, work on the following reflexes:

Autonomic nerves

Lungs/Cardiac

Liver/Spleen

Large intestine

Spine

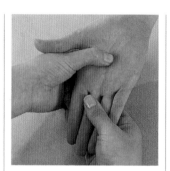

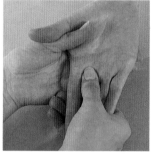

1 Autonomic nerves reflex

 01.00 min

Place your working thumb in the centre of your partner's palm. Apply a little pressure and stimulate with small circles.

2 Lungs/Cardiac reflex

 01.00 min

Place your working thumb between zones 2 and 3. Caterpillar walk to the base of the fingers between the bones. Repeat this between zones 3 and 4 and zones 4 and 5. For the cardiac area, walk from right to left, starting at the finger base and ending at the diaphragm line.

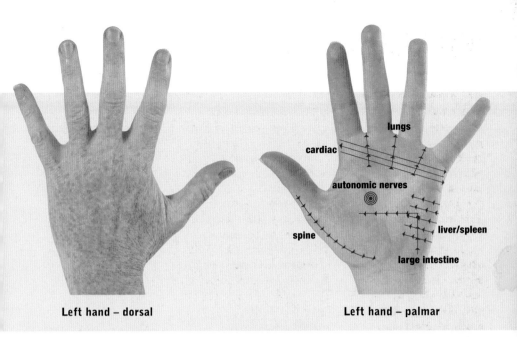

lungs
cardiac
autonomic nerves
spine
liver/spleen
large intestine

Left hand – dorsal

Left hand – palmar

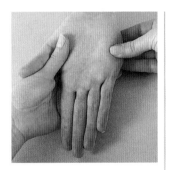

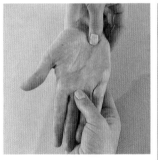

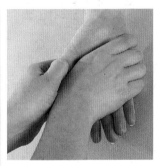

3 Liver (right hand)/Spleen (left hand) reflex

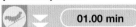 01.00 min

Place your working thumb on the edge of your partner's hand about one thumbprint down from the base of the little finger. Using the caterpillar walk, take three small steps into the hand. Continue in this manner for five lines, finishing just above the wrist.

4 Large intestine reflex

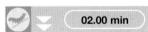 02.00 min

Place your working thumb at the base of zone 4 just above your partner's wrist. Turn your thumbnail so it faces up to the ring finger. Walk up zone 4 until halfway up the hand. Push down and stimulate before turning to walk across the hand, ending up between the webbing.

5 Spine reflex

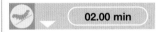 02.00 min

'Shake hands' with your partner. Caterpillar walk along the bone of the thumb from the first to the second joint. Continue to walk along the bone from the second joint to the base of the hand. Stimulate with small circles at each step.

coping with stress

Stress features in all aspects of our lives and can lead to psychological problems such as anxiety and depression, as well as mental and physical problems. Many disorders are directly related to stress and may be made worse by its effects.

If the stress that produces adverse symptoms is not handled properly, more serious illnesses may result. Under prolonged stress, the body is unable to replenish its nutrients quickly, which may make it more vulnerable to disease and slow down healing. Coping with stress is one of the most important uses of hand reflexology. Practising it will help to generally relax the body and allow it to recover.

Using this sequence
Practise this treatment at least once a day in a quiet, stress-free environment. Remember the importance of breathing properly. Taking slow deep breaths throughout the treatment will have a calming effect on the body, and a relaxed body can heal itself.

To help with these conditions, work on the following reflexes:

Hypothalamus

Spine

Lungs

Large intestine

Kidney/Adrenal glands

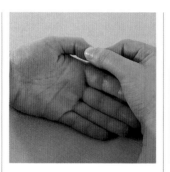

1 Hypothalamus reflex

 01.00 min

Support your thumb on the fingers of one hand. Use your working thumb to stimulate the outside edge of the thumb. Take deep breaths while you are stimulating with small circles.

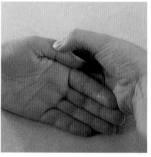

2 Spine reflex

 01.00 min

Cradle one hand in the other. Use your working thumb to caterpillar walk along the bone of the thumb from the first to the second joint. Continue to walk along the bone from the second joint to the base of the hand.

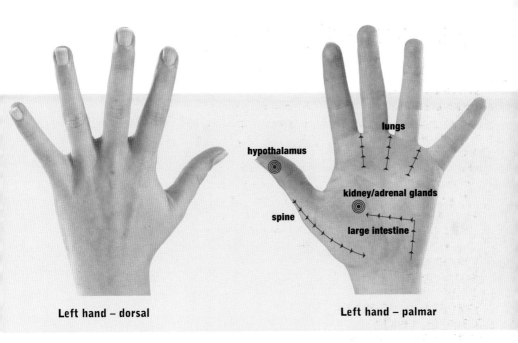

hypothalamus

lungs

kidney/adrenal glands

spine

large intestine

Left hand – dorsal   **Left hand – palmar**

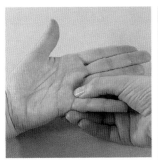

3 Lungs reflex

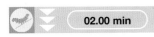
02.00 min

Place your working thumb halfway down the palm of your hand between zones 4 and 5. Apply pressure and caterpillar walk towards the base of the fingers and between the bones. Continue in this manner between zones 3 and 4 and zones 2 and 3.

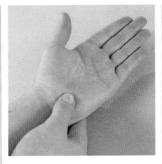

4 Large intestine reflex

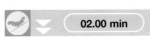
02.00 min

Place your working thumb at the base of zone 4 just above your wrist. Turn your thumbnail so it faces up to the ring finger. Walk up zone 4 until halfway up the hand. Push down and stimulate before turning to walk across the hand, ending up between the webbing.

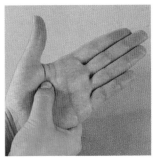

5 Kidney/Adrenal glands reflex

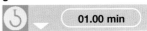
01.00 min

Support one hand in the other. Place your working thumb in the webbing between the thumb and index finger just above the thumb muscle halfway down the hand. Use your thumb to hook into the webbing and apply pressure.

counteracting stress

The body has some basic control mechanisms to counteract everyday stresses. However, if stress is unusually long-lasting or extreme, these control mechanisms can be harmful to the body.

There are three phases of adaptation to stress: alarm, resistance and finally exhaustion. Each phase is controlled by hormones and, since stress can have a disrupting effect on the hormonal system, it can create an excellent breeding ground for illness. Research estimates that stress contributes to 80 per cent of major illnesses, including cardiovascular disease and cancer.

Hand reflexology helps alleviate the effects of stress by inducing deep relaxation, allowing the nervous system to function normally and freeing the body to find its natural balance.

Using this sequence

Practise this treatment at least once a day in a quiet, stress-free environment. Use it in conjunction with the 'Coping with stress' sequence on page 116 to help the body build up its natural defences against disease and cope with the effects of stress.

To help with these conditions, work on the following reflexes:

Head

Pituitary

Occipital bone

Kidney/Adrenal glands

Lymphatics

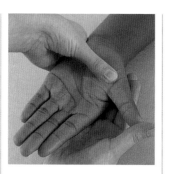

1 Head reflex

 01.00 min

Support your partner's hand. Use your working thumb to walk either down from the tip or up from the base of the thumb. Continue in this manner until you have covered the area. Stimulate with tiny circles at each step.

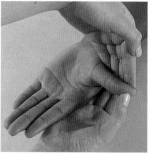

2 Pituitary reflex

 01.00 min

Support your partner's hand in the palm of your hand. Use your working thumb to apply pressure and stimulate the centre of your partner's thumb.

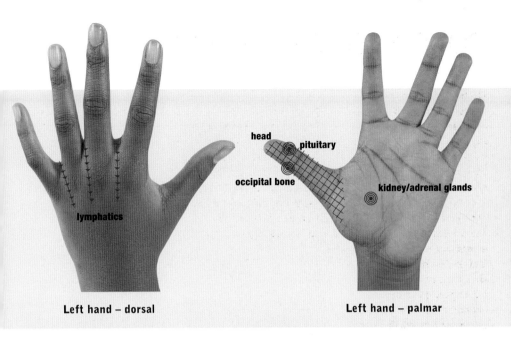

head
pituitary
occipital bone
kidney/adrenal glands
lymphatics

Left hand – dorsal

Left hand – palmar

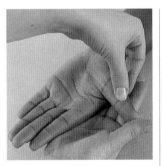

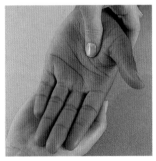

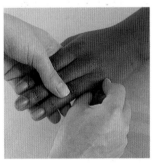

3 Occipital bone reflex

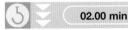 02.00 min

Support your partner's thumb in one hand. Place your working thumb against the first joint of the thumb. Hook up against the bone and stimulate in clockwise or anticlockwise circles.

4 Kidney/Adrenal glands reflex

 01.00 min

Cradle your partner's hand in your hands. Place your working thumb in the webbing between your partner's thumb and index finger just above the thumb muscle halfway down the hand. Use your thumb to hook into the webbing and apply pressure.

5 Lymphatics reflex

 02.00 min

Place your partner's hand palm downward. Place your working index finger and thumb between the bases of the ring and little fingers. Using bird's beak, take tiny steps towards the wrist. Continue in this manner between zones 3 and 4 and zones 2 and 3.

emotional wellbeing

State of mind is closely associated with wellbeing of the body. Negative emotions can show themselves in the body as disease if they are not corrected.

Practise deep breathing whenever you need to take control of your emotions. Inhale deeply with your mouth closed, hold your breath for a few seconds, then exhale slowly through your mouth. Do this while stimulating the solar plexus in the centre of your hand (see page 51) until the tension passes.

Gentle hand reflexology can help us cope with difficult situations that seem to be out of control. It provides a safe way of calming the emotions and has no unpleasant side-effects. A hand reflexology session will provide the quiet time necessary for letting new ideas generate, giving you renewed mental energy and a positive outlook.

Using this sequence
Practise deep breathing throughout the treatment. Use the sequence below as a pick-me-up in the morning, the middle of the day or the late afternoon.

To help with these conditions, work on the following reflexes:

Sinuses

Diaphragm

Neck

Spine

Pineal gland

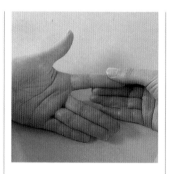

1 Sinuses reflex

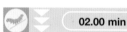
02.00 min

Support the fingers of one hand in the other. Using your working thumb, walk from the tip to the base, or the base to the tip, of one finger. Continue in this manner until you have worked all the fingers. Stimulate with tiny circles at each step.

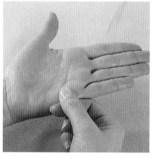

2 Diaphragm reflex

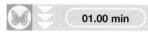
01.00 min

Place your working thumb a third of the way down the palm of your other hand. Use the butterfly movement to walk across the hand from one side to the other.

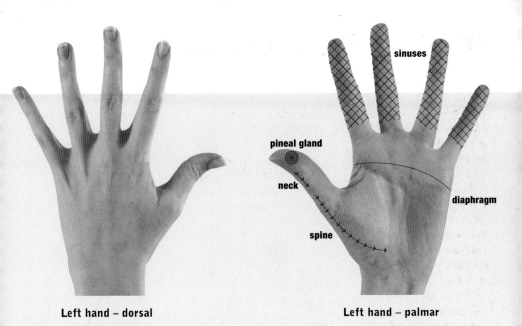

Left hand – dorsal

Left hand – palmar

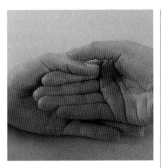

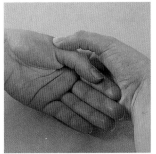

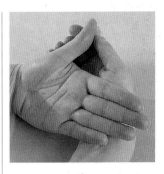

3 Neck reflex

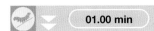 01.00 min

Cradle your thumb in your fingers. Use your working thumb to walk along the bone of the thumb from the first to the second joint. Make seven small steps along the bone, to represent the seven vertebrae in the neck. Stimulate with small circles at each step.

4 Spine reflex

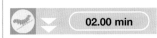 02.00 min

Cradle one hand in the other. Use your working thumb to walk along the bone, starting at the base of the thumb. Make 12 small steps along the bone to the edge of the wrist. Continue along the bone to the base of the hand.

5 Pineal gland reflex

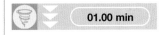 01.00 min

Support your thumb on the fingers of one hand. Use your working thumb to stimulate the inside edge of the centre of your thumb. Take deep breaths while you are stimulating the area with small circles.

nutrients and detoxification

Our supply of nutrients depends not only on what foods and drinks we consume, but on how well our body is able to digest them. A good diet contains a balance of carbohydrates, proteins, fats and vitamins and minerals, while a healthy digestive system ensures that the nutrients they contain are absorbed properly.

Detoxification is the processing and elimination of waste matter from the body. Any illness has a negative effect on how the body handles such wastes. To keep body systems functioning well, you must eat healthily, chew your food well to release the digestive enzymes and drink at least 2 litres (about 4 pints) of water a day.

Using this sequence
This treatment can be used up to three times a day to help revitalize a sluggish digestive system, increase the circulation, aid vitamin and nutrient absorption, and release toxins and waste products so that the body can eliminate them efficiently.

To help with these conditions, work on the following reflexes:

Oesophagus

Gall bladder

Stomach

Liver/Spleen

Large intestine

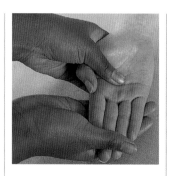

1 Oesophagus reflex

 01.00 min

Place your working thumb halfway down your partner's hand between zones 2 and 3 and walk up between the bones to the bases of the index and middle fingers. Continue in this manner, stimulating with small circles at each step.

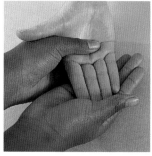

2 Gall bladder reflex

 01.00 min

Place your working thumb on the diaphragm line at the joint at the base of your partner's ring finger. Hook up towards the ring finger and stimulate with tiny circles against the joint.

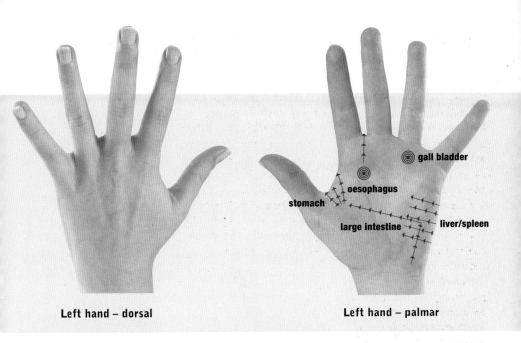

gall bladder

oesophagus

stomach

large intestine

liver/spleen

Left hand – dorsal

Left hand – palmar

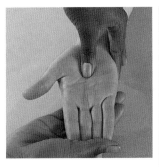

3 Stomach reflex

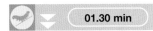
01.30 min

Support your partner's hand. Place your working thumb at the tip of the webbing between the thumb and index finger, then walk to the edge of the hand and return back to your original point. Continue until you have covered the webbing, rather like the spokes of a bicycle wheel.

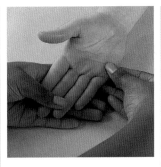

4 Liver (right hand)/Spleen (left hand) reflex

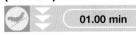
01.00 min

Place your working thumb on the edge of your partner's hand about one thumbprint down from the base of the little finger. Using the caterpillar walk, take three small steps into the hand. Continue in this manner for five lines, finishing just above the wrist.

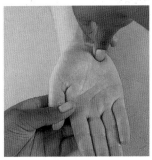

5 Large intestine reflex

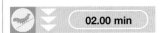
02.00 min

Place your working thumb at the base of zone 4 just above your partner's wrist. Turn your thumbnail so it faces up to the ring finger. Walk up zone 4 until halfway up the hand. Push down and stimulate before turning to walk across the hand, ending up between the webbing.

index

acknowledgements

Louise Keet:
I would like to thank Ziggie and Phoenix Bergman for their unconditional love, St John Freeth Wright for his help and contribution to this book, Marcella Courtfield for always being there with inspiration, Irene Lemos for her great mind, Deborah Dor and MJ Low for their wonderful friendship, Jane McIntosh, Jessica Cowie and Leigh Jones for their expertise and guidance, the Association of Reflexologists, and all the students and graduates of the Central London School of Reflexology for their help and support.

Michael Keet:
I would like to thank Paul Mansell for his drawings of the moves and my dearest lifelong friend Nena Jukes for her advice and wisdom. I would like to thank my granddad Stan Richards for his devotion and love, my dear friends Patrick Thomas and Roz Pendelbury,

and a special thankyou to my son Phoenix for being born. I would also like to thank Atsuko Kamiji at the Yokohama School of Reflexology and the therapists and staff at our school Le Sport in St Lucia.

Picture Acknowledgements:
Special Photography: © **Octopus Publishing Group Limited**/Peter Pugh-Cook.
Other photography: **Werner Forman Archive** 10. **Getty Images**/Julie Toy 19. **Paolo Scremin /Oxford Expedition to Egypt** 11. **Wellcome Trust, Medical Photographic Library** 16-17.

Executive Editor: **Jane McIntosh**
Editor: **Leanne Bryan**
Executive Art Editor: **Karen Sawyer**
Designer: **Peter Gerrish**
Illustrator: **Kate Nardoni/Cactus Design**
Production Controller: **Nosheen Shan**
Medical Consultant: **Dr Michael Apple**